What is Healing and Growth? Thoughts from Freud

What is Healing and Growth? Thoughts from Freud

By

Anthony F. Badalamenti

Cambridge
Scholars
Publishing

What is Healing and Growth? Thoughts from Freud

By Anthony F. Badalamenti

This book first published 2021

Cambridge Scholars Publishing

Lady Stephenson Library, Newcastle upon Tyne, NE6 2PA, UK

British Library Cataloguing in Publication Data
A catalogue record for this book is available from the British Library

ISBN (10): 1-5275-6794-X
ISBN (13): 978-1-5275-6794-8

TABLE OF CONTENTS

PREFACE

Healing and Growth are the prime goals of any form of psychotherapy, making this a likely reason for the emphasis on technique and method in its history. Much of healing and growth is easily seen, and certainly enjoyed, by both patient and therapist, giving research into its nature a back seat to the primary goal of relieving suffering and promoting growth. At the same time it seems likely that the advances garnered in more than a century of work in various modalities should contain hints at the nature of healing and growth. This expresses the perspective taken in this book with respect to the works of Sigmund Freud.

Like his contemporaries and those who came after him, he was looking for an understanding of what causes psychological suffering with the hope and anticipation that such understanding would lead to new and better methods of treatment. His works built to a model for how the personality both develops and functions in health and unhealth. He strongly felt that understanding pathology, which can result in extreme expressions of component parts of the personality, makes it easier to see and understand how the personality functions in a state of health. His writings emphasize the relief of symptoms and gains in the power to adapt as outcomes of successful psychotherapy, but rarely would he comment on the nature of healing and growth itself, that is its process dynamics.

Yet he left a trail of crumbs, so to speak, in his writings that is rich in implicit clues as to how healing and growth take place. Like his psychoanalytic model itself, such hints do not build to a compete representation of the process, but they form a good start.

INTRODUCTION

Anyone seeking psychotherapy is suffering with an emotional problem of some sort and usually senses that there are better ways to deal with life. The negative feelings, or symptoms, involved are usually varieties of anxiety and depression, including feelings of panic, confusion and agitation. In some instances flooding is the most distressing symptom, without reference to the nature of the feelings that the patient is flooded with. In all instances the negative feelings are a part of a personality configuration that results in poor adaptation in some parts of life and often in a sense of being out of sorts. These are surface descriptions that can only hint at what an emotional problem is, this being a precursor to beginning to deal with the issues of treatment and resolution.

If an emotional problem is regarded as an approximate term for a neurosis, then the latter's defining feature of developmental arrest becomes useful in defining what an emotional problem is. A developmental arrest means that part of the personality has failed to fully mature, implying limited powers of adaptation, and more subtly, implying a neurosis, psychosis or borderline disorder. The fact that a developmental arrest implies that parts of the personality are still functioning at an infantile level is most easily seen in neurosis where they contrast strongly with the healthily functioning, mature parts of the personality. The adjective infantile here means that, in the case of neurosis, the point of arrest is usually between the ages of two and five, in the borderline case earlier and in the case of psychosis, still earlier.

When a child's environment presents stresses too strong for its young and growing personality to manage an arrest will follow. The underlying principle is that nature wants to safeguard the child's ability to keep growing psychologically. When overly strong stresses tax the child beyond its capacity to adapt nature creates defenses whose purpose is to isolate the child's unmanageably strong emotional responses from the rest of its personality, especially from its consciousness. This preserves the ability of the rest of the child's personality to continue to grow. For example, if the father of a girl around the age of two or three fails to give her sufficient emotional attention, then the child's frustration will lead to rage reactions, and if these are too much for the little girl to manage then a defense like repression may result; if the stresses are strong enough then a more primitive defense such as a reaction formation may enter. Within childhood the invocation of defenses can be regarded as a positive adaptation because, while limiting maturation of the personality overall, it enables the rest of it to continue to flower and also spares the child consciously suffering overly strong feelings such as rage, guilt and helplessness.

Once set in place defenses continue to operate, from childhood to the adult state unless the child's environment ceases to be overly stressful, an unlikely event in most cases. Whether regarded as a positive adaptation or not in childhood, the outcome is a neurosis because what is blocked by defenses continues to exist in an early form that continues to struggle against defenses to resume its maturation, an event that requires access to consciousness and to parts of the personality that have access to consciousness. Where there is pathology this fails and the result is that the energy of the blocked emotions becomes expressed in the derivative form of symptoms. That is, what nature intended to mature into expressed powers of adaptation can only express itself in the maladaptive form of symptoms. In the above example, the child's blocked rage could find expression in such symptoms as oppositional behavior, negativism, or overtly destructive behavior such as breaking items of value. To make matters worse, the child's personality will respond with guilt to the presence of its rage and this will reach consciousness as anxiety and possibly depression.

The goal of analysis, whether in childhood or later, is to free what is blocked so that it can resume the growth intended for it by nature from the outset. This is done in psychoanalysis, as well as in dynamic forms of therapy, mostly by the work of interpretation, the idea being to first create a cognitive awareness of how one is unconsciously working against oneself emotionally and to open ever larger paths from cognitive to emotional awareness. This is a form of healing because the process liberates blocked drives seeking access to consciousness and other parts of the personality that can link with consciousness, enabling them to flower once again. This is part of what Freud had in mind when he referred to the work of psychoanalysis as making the unconscious conscious. It is also healing in the sense that the interpretive process, when successful, ends the expression of what is blocked as symptoms and leads to a transformation of its expression to the burgeoning of healthy adaptive powers for life.

The above is a broad brush description of healing and growth that points to the main direction of this book. What it is that heals, what it is that grows and what inner structural changes occur, and how all these take place are among the specifics to be filled in.

Freud felt that in order for a psychological explanation to be complete it must touch upon structural, dynamic and economic aspects of what is being explained. The structural components in his model are the id, ego and superego, where the id is the seat of instinctual tendencies or drives, the ego is the executive part of the personality that does the work of meeting the demands of the id, ego, superego and reality, and the superego is essentially the same as what is understood as conscience, but based on the internalization of parental and cultural values. In the original German Freud used the words das Es, meaning the It (to emphasize the primitive nature of the Id), the word das Ich translating as the I (to emphasize the executive character of the ego) and the word das Uber-Ich meaning the over I (to emphasize both the judgmental and rewarding roles of the superego). The Latin words, id, ego and superego mean it, I and over/above the I, respectively. These words entered when Freud's writings were translated into English at a time when it was still fashionable to use Latin in medical contexts.

The dynamic part of the explanation presents how the components of the personality interact with one another as well as how sub components within each component interact. Freud added to these structural and dynamic requirements the need for an explanation to account for how energy is utilized in the personality, this being the economic perspective.

The present description of healing and growth will touch upon the above three dimensions. However, its main emphasis will be on how the primary and secondary processes evolve within psychotherapy. The *primary* process describes mostly *affective* events in the id and cognitive ones in the lower ego and id/ego boundary. The *secondary* process describes mostly *cognitive* events, in the ego, including the lower ego close to the ego/id boundary. In Freud's model the primary process governs weakly differentiated perceptions as seen in dreams and symptoms, but the secondary governs highly differentiated ones as seen in the real work of adaptation, including psychotherapy

Freud and his tradition have discussed aspects of healing and growth. Freud emphasized that healing and growth see a person outgrow the pleasure principle in favor of the reality principle, meaning that the early tendency to recoil away from unpleasure is slowly replaced by tolerance of the unpleasure when enough reality sense has emerged within the person to see that eventual pleasure will result. He also emphasized his familiar quip that where there was id there will be ego, referring to his view that the ego grows out of the id as something of an interface with both reality and the superego, the one presenting actual opportunities and constraints from the world and the other presenting ethical or moral constraints arising from within. Freud saw the major work of therapy as the use of interpretation to undo defenses that stand in the way of healing and growth in these and other senses. One of these other senses is the decreasing use of primary process functioning and the increasing use of secondary process functioning, major hallmarks of healing and growth.

A major organizing theme of what follows is that while the work of psychotherapy brings about structural, dynamic and economic changes in the ego, id and superego, all such changes are most easily seen in how the work of therapy moves the primary and secondary processes toward healthier, more adaptive functioning. Freud's narrative repeatedly gives qualitative descriptions of the primary process that stop short of the exact formulations of physics, an unsurprising event given his roots in determinism. These descriptions will be of considerable use in realizing the goal in the above organizing theme.

It will be useful to begin with a discussion of the inner workings of Freud as a researcher, that is, the relation of his personality and temperament to how he carried out his psychological research.

CHAPTER 1

FREUD'S PERSONALITY

It often happens that a person reading Freud for the first time feels surprise, even astonishment, at his ability to see the things he describes. He clearly had an unusual gift from nature for understanding psychological relationships but some of his ability is made understandable with knowledge of his personality because he also had ordinary gifts and character traits that very likely would not have led to his discoveries without his unusual gift

He described himself as an obsessional personality, a disorder that he studied thoroughly not only because of his findings in his self analysis but also because much of his practice consisted of obsessionals. Among his findings was their concern with issues of morality, defined more by their own subjective sense of right and wrong than by their ambient culture. He found this trait so thorough going and prominent in obsessionals that he often said of them that they maintained a private religion, more because of the great attention they gave to living within their way and to not violating it than to the frequent presence of ritualistic behaviors among them. Obsessionals have their individual, very personal, standards of integrity and their well being depends strongly of meeting them. That this was true of Freud is expressed in the quotation below. The inserted English translations of the French appear as footnotes in the original:

"Some years later, at one of Charcot's evening receptions, I happened to be standing near the great teacher at a moment when he appeared to be telling Brouardel a very interesting story about something that had happened during his day's work. I hardly heard the beginning, but gradually my attention was seized by what he was talking of: a young married couple from a distant country in the East – the woman, a severe sufferer, the man either impotent or exceedingly awkward. 'Tachez donc,' (Go on trying!) I heard Charcot repeating, 'je vous assure, vous y arriverez.' (I promise you, you'll succeed.) Brouardel, who spoke less loudly, must have expressed his astonishment that symptoms like the wife's could have been produced by such circumstances. For Charcot suddenly broke out with great animation: 'Mais, dons des cas pariels c'est toujours la chase genitale toujours...

toujours...toujours'; (But in this sort of case it's always a question of the genitals – always, always, always.) And he crossed his arms over his stomach, hugging himself and jumping up and down on his toes several times in his own characteristically lively way. I know that for a moment I was almost paralyzed with amazement and said to myself: 'Well, but if he knows that, why does he never say so?'" (Freud, 2001, Vol XIV, 13-14)

Freud was about twenty nine at the time, a young physician who expected even Charcot, whom he greatly admired as his mentor and for his research into hypnotism at the Salpetriere in Paris, to meet his own standards of scientific integrity. There are many other similar quotes where physicians privately talk of sexual causality in the neuroses but publicly deny it. Most such statements were made at a time when Freud's conviction of an empirical basis for sexual causality was at odds both with the spirit of the times and the medical community, but such trends did not deter him. The need to understand the inner workings of nature, especially in the biological sense, was strong in him, a need that gained strength from the obsessional trait in him. His inquiring ways were there from the beginning but their first object was religion.

He was disappointed by what religions, including his own Judaism, had to offer, He found them to be without foundation, often superstitious in nature and unsatisfying as sources of understanding for human behavior, nature and life in general. Most especially they lacked the empirical, verifiable basis that science offered. The rigorous methods and standards of science appealed to both his hunger for knowledge and to his need for integrity in the offerings. There was more to Freud's emphasis on honest inquiry than his obsessional trend to insist on integrity. Within his model an obsessional is developmentally arrested in the anal stage because of rage reactions to environmental stresses that are too strong for the person's young psyche to deal with consciously. The psyche automatically creates reaction formations, a very strong way to defend against the rage, to keep it away from consciousness as well as from parts of the psyche that easily connect with it. As noted earlier, the outcome is something of a deal with the devil because the reaction formation seals off a part of the psyche, preserving the ability of the rest of it to keep flowering as well as sparing the child's consciousness the painful task of dealing with overly strong feelings, but it also results in the defended against part becoming unable to develop further in most ways because of its being sealed off from most of the rest of personality and its vital energies.

In terms of pain, suffering and limited growth potential, the stakes are high in the obsessional defense. The risk of experiencing strong, if not overwhelming, anxiety associated with the given stresses continues through the anal stage and results in the reaction formation creating ever more elaborate and convoluted ways of keeping the rage blocked, these forming the obsessional's system. The need to insist on integrity was part of Freud's system, and like all such systems, it had a driven quality that belied it. Thematically this led to a joining of the need for knowledge with the need for honesty. Early on this had a neurotic coloring but with time he put aside his disappointment with religion and held onto the positive experience of his natural curiosity, making the joining of his need for knowledge with his need for honesty an increasingly healthy and trustworthy pursuit of knowledge. That is, with time his need for integrity in the pursuit of knowledge became less driven, approximating ever more to a healthy, strong but tempered interest in the verifiable findings of science. It is likely that Freud, as a child, felt that his parents were being deceitful with him, a thing he often reported on with his patients as resulting in a later driven quest for reliable knowledge. It is also likely that Freud, before committing to study medicine, considered studying law because of its connection with rights and integrity.

As noted, Freud continued his investigation into the causes of psychological suffering, or pathology, undeterred by both his zeitgeist and his colleagues' opposition to his ideas. This calls for stamina and again touches upon Freud's view of himself as an obsessional. Among the character traits associated with arrest in the anal stage are stubbornness and defiance, both sources of stamina for him in his early efforts to hold his own against an environment that was hostile to his findings and often to him personally. As an adult his defiance did not tend to find expression as contempt for authority, as it usually does, but more as contempt for those who disagreed with him. To some degree he sublimated these trends into healthy perseverance with his research and, at a more conscious level, into self sustaining confidence, all this adding to his healthy curiosity about the riddle of the neuroses and pathology in general.

Curiosity was not the only healthy trait in him related to his life's work. He was deeply interested in advancing civilization. As a young man he often expressed his wish to contribute to the well being of mankind, a healthy wish living side by side with his cynical and often suspicious view of the human race. This wish often manifested in individual acts of kindness and compassion, sometimes offered at his own expense in money and not just in time and effort. He was humanitarian despite his often dark view of life.

The traits cited thus far – integrity in research and elsewhere, love of science, stubbornness and defiance, curiosity, wishing to contribute to civilization and being humanitarian – do not account for Freud's unusual ability to sense psychological meaning. They fail even when taken together because such trait clustering often occurs in people not noted for their giftedness. The missing piece in accounting for his contributions involves the specific nature of his gifts and this enters in a puzzling way because of the fact that his early interests were limited to medicine and his specialty in neurology. He showed no psychological leanings until events in his practice and research drove him to ask questions of a psychological nature. He showed signs of high intelligence in his childhood and early life, but signs of giftedness did not appear until he was about thirty years old. It follows that his gifts did not flower until later in his life or until they were cued forward by his work, or perhaps a mixture of the two.

A clear presentation of the specific nature of his gifts, and their relation to the cited personality traits, first requires some narrative on the distinction between feelings and emotions. Putting aside the subjective sensations that are part of experiencing feelings, the major function of feelings is to inform or provide information. For example, a person might report having a bad feeling about a circumstance without knowing why, reflecting an unconscious perception of something negative or unfavorable about the circumstance. Freud's idea that neurotic anxiety has a signal function is another example of an unconscious perception leading to a feeling that informs of danger. It can also happen that the reasons for the feeling are also conscious as in someone driving and seeing a road hazard in the distance or, along positive lines, a person feeling delighted at the unexpected sight of a rainbow. The unconscious perceptions that generate a feeling that informs are intuitive in nature and form a rapid means of making decisions which, if made on the basis of a fully studied conscious evaluation, would require too much time to be adaptive.

The perceptions and inner processing that precede feelings can be both conscious and unconscious. For example, a female who has been listening without attention to background music may hear advertising for dance lessons just at a time in her life when she has been thinking of getting better at dancing. The emergent feelings of interest, if not excitement, that result proceed from both conscious and unconscious perceptions. Similar things can be said for the onset of moods.

The fact that unconscious perceptions lead to feelings that provide adaptively useful information for consciousness raises the question as to why conscious perceptions would not lead to the same event because in the latter case one is already informed. Feelings do more than inform, they also lead to states of arousal that are preparatory for action, this being a hallmark of emotion as well as one reason why most people use the terms feeling and emotion interchangeably. The state of arousal results in new conscious feelings that tell on it, whether the originating context is formed by unconscious or by conscious perceptions.

The origin of the word emotion reveals much of its meaning and how this differs from the meaning of feeling. The root of emotion is the Latin verb emovere, meaning to move out. The word emotion comes from emotus, the participle of emovere, and means having been moved out. An emotion is a state of arousal that is meant to result in an expressed action. When the action is inhibited by pathology or other causes, the aroused state discharges as a symptom such as anxiety, agitation or altered body states. The event sequence with an emotion is first the presentation of some adaptive need, followed by body changes that mobilize for action, followed by feelings that inform consciousness of the aroused state. The presenting need usually arises from without but can arise from within, as with hormonal change, the undoing of defenses leading to a liberation of once blocked drives which then reach for expression, and so on. Body changes, such as elevated breathing and heart rates and muscular tension quickly enter awareness as physical sensations that prepare for action. The subjective feelings stir cognitive processing that leads to identifying what adaptive actions might be taken. To take a familiar example, a male sees a female whom he would very much like to connect with. A rush of pleasant body and feeling sensations follow, the former to prepare for action, the latter to hint at how to make a connection with her. Emotion enters in the prior sentence with the goal of an expressed action crafted to hopefully create success.

Feelings may or may not lead to emotional states. A person may feel in the mood to sing but may also fail to do so because of inhibitions. However, emotional states are always attended by feelings that alert awareness to their presence. In the prior example there are feelings that lead to emotional arousal but not strongly enough to result in action, the end state of emotion. In summary form, feelings inform and emotions prepare for action with the caveat that feelings are a connecting link from informing to mobilizing for emotion.

Obsessionals have insufficient contact with some of their feelings and with some parts of their emotional system, making for limited or weak sensing of some feelings and emotions in others. However, where an obsessional is not blocked, there is adequate sensing. Paradoxically, Freud was an obsessional who had a remarkable ability to empathize with the feelings and emotions of others, except for his admitted limitation in his ability to do so with aspects of females. This discussion is building to a description of the exact nature of a fortuitous gift in Freud for understanding psychological meanings. Commentary on some of his own words will be helpful.

The word feeling occurs four times in the quote below:

"We remain on the surface so long as we are dealing only with memories and ideas. What is alone of value in mental life is rather the feelings. No mental forces are significant unless they possess the characteristic of arousing feelings. Ideas are only repressed because they are associated with the release of feelings which ought not to occur. It would be more correct to say that repression acts upon feelings, but we can only be aware of these in their association with ideas." (Freud, 2001, Vol IX, 48-49)

As expected the narrative refers to memories and ideas but only in their capacity to arouse feelings. When Freud indicates that only feelings are of value he is referring to them as sources of information on the patient's inner state, to both the patient and to the analyst, as revealed in his emphasis on the work of repression being not so much to block ideas as to block the feelings they evoke.

Freud gives some biographical information below that arose in a dream he had already interpreted but not to his satisfaction:

"At this point I shall once more take up the interpretation of a dream which we have already found instructive – the dream of my friend R. being my uncle...We have followed its interpretation to the point of recognizing clearly as one of its motives my wish to be appointed to a professorship; and we explained the affection I felt in the dream for my friend R. as a product of opposition and revolt against the slanders upon my two colleagues which were contained in the dream thoughts. The dream was one of my own; I may therefore continue its analysis by saying that my feelings were not yet satisfied by the solution that had so far been reached." (Freud, 2001, Vol IV, 191-192)

His lack of satisfaction is in the words "my feelings were not yet satisfied by the solution that had so far been reached," meaning that a feeling arose within him from an unidentified inner sense that his interpretation up to the given point was incomplete. The same sense of an inner feeling informing on an intuitive perception of incompleteness is in the quote below.

"At the conclusion of my earlier lecture on anxiety I myself expressed the opinion that, although these various findings of our inquiry were not mutually contradictory, somehow they did not fit in with one another. Anxiety, it seems, in so far as it is an affective state, is the reproduction of an old event which brought a threat of danger; anxiety serves the purposes of self-preservation and is a signal of a new danger; it arises from libido that has in some way become unemployable and it also arises during the process of repression; it is replaced by the formation or a symptom, is, as it were, psychically bound – one has a feeling that something is missing here which would bring all these pieces together into a whole." (Freud, 2001, Vol XXII, 84)

That the role of feeling is more in the nature of a messenger of intuitive processing than the intuition itself is expressed below.

"...She complained at this moment of some frightful pains, and made one last desperate effort to reject the explanation: it was not true, I had talked her into it, it *could* not be true, she was incapable of such wickedness, she could never forgive herself for it. It was easy to prove to her that what she herself had told me admitted of no other interpretation. But it was a long time before my two pieces of consolation – that we are not responsible for our feelings, and that her behaviour, the fact that she had fallen ill in these circumstances, was sufficient evidence of her moral character– it was a long time before these consolations of mine made any impression on her." (Freud, Vol II, 157)

Although the phrase "that we are not responsible for our feelings" has a moralizing tone meant to assuage the patient's anxiety, it has relevant implications elsewhere. Freud's other point here is that feelings arise on their own, uninvited and uncaused by either consciousness or volition. This relates to powers of unconscious perception and inference that precede the emergence of feelings. Freud's inner reliance on such powers is in the next quote:

"...We are engaged in investigating the technique of jokes as shown in examples; and we should therefore be certain that the examples we have chosen are really genuine jokes.... We have no criterion at our disposal before our investigation has given us one. Linguistic usage is untrustworthy and itself needs to have its justification examined. In coming to our decision we can base ourselves on nothing but a certain '*feeling*', which we may interpret as meaning that the decision is made in our judgment in accordance with particular criteria that are not yet accessible to our knowledge." (Freud, 2001, Vol VIII, 61).

The basis for Freud's inner reliance on such powers is made more explicit in the next two quotes:

"...If so, however, we may safely assume that no generation is able to conceal any of its more important mental processes from its successor. For psychoanalysis has shown us that everyone possesses in his unconscious mental activity an apparatus which enables him to interpret other people's reactions, that is, to undo the distortions which other people have imposed on the expression of their feelings. An unconscious understanding such as this of all the customs, ceremonies and dogmas left behind by the original relation to the father may have made it possible for later generations to take over their heritage of emotions." (Freud, 2001, Vol XIII, 159)

"...She now did all she could to prevent her husband from guessing that she had fallen ill owing to the frustration of which he was the cause. But I have good reason for asserting that everyone posses in his own unconscious an instrument with which he can interpret the utterances of the unconscious in other people. Her husband understood, without any admission or explanation on her part, what his wife's anxiety meant, he felt hurt, without showing it, and in his turn reacted neurotically by – for the first time – failing in sexual intercourse with her." (Freud, 2001, Vol XII, 320)

The term apparatus in the first quote and instrument in the second refer to ego capacities for both perception and for forming inferences based on perception, mostly but not entirely unconscious in the observer. The quotes thus far are intended to reveal Freud's empathic dependence upon feelings to arrive at information on the patient's inner world, this being mostly of an emotional character. Thus far, the quotes do not hint at how he saw the relation of feeling to emotion and vice versa, nor do they hint at his understanding of the relation of empathy to both feeling and emotion.

Here is a first expression of his idea on the relationship between emotion and feeling:

"It is true that 'unconscious ideas' never, or only rarely and with difficulty, enter waking thought, but they influence it. They do so, first, through their consequences – when, for instance, a patient is tormented by a hallucination which is totally unintelligible and senseless, but whose meaning and motivation become clear under hypnosis. Further, they influence association by making certain ideas more vivid than they would have been if they had not been thus reinforced from the unconscious. So particular groups of ideas constantly force themselves on the patient with a certain amount of compulsion and he is obliged to think of them...Again, unconscious ideas govern the patient's emotional tone, his state of feelings." (Freud, 2001, Vol II, 237)

All but the last line of the quoted material refer to how unconscious ideas forge emotional connections with other parts of the personality, this leading to states of arousal as indicated by the words influence, vivid and compulsion. The position that unconscious ideas govern the patient's emotional tone and his state of feelings expresses how feelings arise from emotional states to inform the person of their presence. The process of emotional states leading to the creation of feelings to inform is explicitly stated below:

> "At the time at which I was attributing to sexuality this important part in the production of the *simple* neuroses, I was still faithful to a purely psychological theory in regard to the *psychoneuroses* – a theory in which the sexual factor was regarded as no more significant than any other emotional source of feeling." (Freud, 2001, Vol VII, 272)

Emotions lead to states of arousal, creating energy meant to be spent in actions that fulfil the associated emotional need, whether healthy or not. The words below refer explicitly to emotional states leading to a need for discharge via action of various kinds.

> "In the first place, it must be emphasized that Breuer's patient, in almost all her pathogenic situations, was obliged to *suppress* a powerful emotion instead of allowing its discharge in the appropriate signs of emotion, words or actions....Quite apart from this, a certain portion of our mental excitation is normally directed along the paths of somatic innervation and produces what we know as an 'expression of the emotions'." (Freud, 2001, Vol XIV, 17-18)

The phrase "a certain portion of our mental excitation is normally directed along the paths of somatic innervation" addresses how emotions, as impelling toward action, lead to bodily arousal, including the familiar facial and other body expressions of an emotional state.

The ten quotations of Freud are meant to create a sense for how his mind and emotional system operated when working to make sense of his patients' inner states, whether understood as feelings or emotions. It is clear that there is more emphasis on the use of feelings than of emotions in these quotations, a thing that is true in general. In fact, in the 5079 pages of Freud's collected works, the word feel and related words such as feeling, felt and so on occur 2369 times, whereas the word emotion and related words occurs 595 times.[1] The ratio of these numbers is 3.98 or essentially 4. It must be said that the fact that there are 8 feeling quotes and 2 emotion quotes above, giving the same ratio, was noted only after the quotations were selected. What's more the decision to count the

---

[1] The cited numbers were found using Adobe search commands on Ivan Smith's "Freud – Complete Works."

number of occurrences cited arose in the process of searching for relevant quotations.

This leads to a formulation of Freud's unusual capacity to sense psychological meaning. When dealing with patients' narratives Freud would experience, as any interested listener would, emotional resonance with each of them. The joint effect of the narrative, its expressed emotion and whatever bodily expression attended it, would result in an emotional state in him that repeated much of the patients' emotional states.[2] His consciousness was informed of the presence and meaning of his resonant emotional states by the feelings that they sired. This is the same point any person observing another would reach and, by itself, does not distinguish Freud from others. In the early part of Freud's era, when psychoanalytic concepts were yet to be formed, someone observing a patient would be not able to move past a feeling based intuition of the meaning of what was observed toward a concept that could reveal its meaning in a literally verbal way, this being a sign of a full conscious understanding of the kind that Freud's work was building towards.

Freud was far more able than most others to let his feelings communicate their meanings to him. This was a two sided process with him. On the one side was a rich openness to experiencing most of his feelings and on the other an intellect capable, in more than one sense, of apprehending their meaning, Greatest among these senses was his ability to let his feelings invite forward into his consciousness those concepts that would naturally associate with the given feelings, this being a gift of nature. His understanding did not stop at the level of nonverbal intuition but, enabled by this gift, he could formulate their meanings in words. The growth of his insights proceeded in a like manner with his self analysis with the proviso that there was no need for empathic resonance to arrive at the emotions and feelings of concern. It similarly applied to his insights culled from casual observation of life with people's ordinary behaviors versus patients in sessions.[3]

His use of this gift was facilitated by the traits cited earlier: – integrity in research and elsewhere, love of science, stubbornness and defiance, curiosity, wishing to contribute to civilization and being humanitarian.

Freud naively expected the medical community of his time to welcome his findings but was roundly disappointed. What's more, word of the

---

[2] The cautious wording on bodily expressions enters because Freud was not in a physical position to look at his patients most of the time.
[3] There are numerous examples of such observations in his works "The Psychopathology of Everyday Life" and "Jokes and Their Relation to the Unconscious."

nature of his findings on sexuality, aggression and unconscious mental life was not only unwelcome to the culture of his day, but also led to acrimony directed at him outside the medical community. The outcome of his disappointment was that his stubborn and defiant way was fuelled by his certainty of his findings, this leading to his continuing his research into the neuroses and mental health in general with renewed vigor. He often referred to this era of his life, the late nineteenth century, as one of splendid isolation. His morale was further lifted by his strong curiosity regarding the nature and origin of psychopathology as well as his love of science. The matter of his colleagues not finding value in his results offended his sense of honesty and integrity, a thing that would amplify his defiance and stubbornness. The same applies to his wish to contribute to civilization and relieve human suffering because, wanting and expecting his colleagues to endorse and use his results when they failed to do so, further offended his sense of integrity. Simultaneously his need to make a living and care for his growing family was an obvious source of motivation for holding the course. Last but far from least was Freud's driven ambition, the wish to make a major contribution to science and to become famous, this and all the above feeding and sustaining his commitment to continue his line of research however unwelcome it might be to others whose opinion he valued. These considerations apply mostly to Freud before he began to gain acceptance in the early twentieth century but do remain in place for the sequel because opposition, though diminishing, was still present for the rest of his life.

A picture of a driven researcher with a special gift emerges. One part of Freud's gift for psychological understanding was his ability to use his resonant feelings to understand the meaning of a patient's emotional state. The other, and perhaps unique part, was his ability to have his feelings evoke well formed – verbalizable – concepts of their meaning and hence the meaning of the patient's inner experience.

There is not yet much hinting at how this bears on clarifying the meaning of healing and growth except in the hope that this material will give the reader some sense of Freud's experience when working and struggling to find meaning in his patients' narratives and the expressed emotions associated with them. The next chapter will discuss how he arrived at psychological research, an interesting point because that is not where he started nor is it where his initial intentions were.

CHAPTER 2

THE WISH TO CURE

When Freud began his medical studies at the University of Vienna in 1873, at age seventeen there was little, if any, of the psychologist in him. He was fascinated by his studies and by his third year his dominating interest in research asserted itself with a project aimed at resolving a question about eels dating back to Aristotle. To resolve whether there is such a thing as a male eel Freud set about dissecting the gonads of several hundred of them. His findings were not conclusive but the vignette tells on the nature of his medical interest. His yen for research asserted itself again some three after this with his work on the use of gold chloride to stain nerve tissue. In the same time frame, he was stimulated by reports of increased stamina in Indians ingesting coca leaf, and this led to his studying the therapeutic properties of cocaine in the mid 1880's. He found it provided some relief for cardiac problems, neurasthenia (emotional or nervous fatigue) and indigestion, among other applications, including anesthesia. He used it to relive his own symptoms of depression and anxiety. Although he was never addicted to it, he was addicted to tobacco, smoking about twenty cigars a day, in part to improve his concentration.

He studied in the departments of psychiatry, dermatology, childhood diseases and others to round out his training but his dominating interest converged on neurology. He was quite satisfied with his world of research even though he scarcely had enough money to meet basic expenses and often had to accept money from his father to help him stay afloat. He might have continued living and working this way indefinitely had he not fallen in love with Martha Bernays. The event gave him firsthand experience with how lovers idolize their beloveds, a point he would eventually write about. Eventually the practical need to earn enough money to marry and have a family with Martha pressed Freud into an unhappy corner because he never wanted to become a physician with a practice but, rather, wanted to remain a physician doing medical research, especially in neurology. Both his love of Martha and of research won the day with his decision to build a practice while maintaining academic connections. They were engaged in 1882 and married in 1886.

He would become a practicing neurologist. The most eminent neurologist of that time was Jean Martin Charcot at the Salpetriere in Paris, the institute where Pinel in the century before this time worked to introduce more humane methods of treatment for the afflicted. Freud was awarded a stipend amounting to far less than he needed to go to Paris and lodge there while studying under Charcot but he made up the needed differences more with enthusiastic resolution than with practicality.

Freud was delighted with his studies under Charcot, finding him a dedicated researcher and a conscientious worker with high standards of scientific integrity and compassion. He formed a close relationship with Charcot, often accompanying him on his rounds at the Salpetriere to learn as much as he could from the man he regarded as his mentor. He was quite impressed with how carefully prepared each of Charcot's lectures was, often referring to them as individual masterpieces of preparation. Charcot was using hypnotism to induce hysterical symptoms and his lectures featured live demonstrations of this. Young Freud was fairly well stunned by what he saw and for a variety of reasons. For one, Charcot's work legitimized hysteria as a bona fide disorder, at least among the French, moving neurology and the times past regarding it as a form of malingering or pretence created for reasons of convenience or personal gain. For another, Freud identified with Charcot's struggle against the criticism of his contemporaries, these being based on Charcot's classification of hysterical symptoms as being no more than a replication of medieval efforts to classify forms of demonic possession.

Charcot's greatest effect on Freud was to move him toward a new way of thinking about neurologic disorders, an effect that worked on him for a very long time, and resulting in his lifelong gratitude to Charcot for setting him on a new direction. Freud quickly saw that Charcot's work implied that ideas could be at the bottom of hysterical symptoms. He also quickly saw that Charcot's work implied that unconscious processes could be operative in the etiology of hysteria. Charcot himself brought these two trains of thought together with his proposal of traumatic etiology for hysteria, and the general principle of traumatic etiology stayed with Freud forever after, as evidenced by his later writings.

The concept of unconscious mental activity was part of Freud's Zeitgeist and he certainly did not invent the idea. Freud's contribution to the idea of unconscious mental activity would be to discover some of its principles of operation. His time with Charcot, approximately five months in Paris, was part of the beginning of Freud's turn to psychological thinking, though it is unlikely that he realized it at the time. Freud's admiration and gratitude for Charcot survived subsequent research that put some of Charcot's findings in question. What lived on in Freud were both Charcot's openness and method, the latter strongly emphasizing that an investigator must look at his data many times over until it spoke its meanings to him, this advice appealing to Freud's gift for seeing what meanings his feelings were giving him.

Another important part of Freud's turn to psychological thinking was his association with Joseph Breuer, a Viennese physician – not a neurologist – fourteen years his elder. His work with Breuer was far more therapeutic and clinical in nature than with Charcot. The two had a close friendship based on shared medical interest and also included Breuer helping Freud in times of financial stress. They jointly authored Studies in Hysteria, where the treatment of a twenty one year old female hysteric, dubbed Anna O is described. Among her many symptoms were paralysis of three limbs, disturbed vision and speech, hallucinations, double personality and inability to eat. Although her native tongue was German she could, at that time, speak only English and when asked to read from a book written in a language she knew, such as French, she would recite in English.

Her actual name was Bertha Pappenheim and this is noted because she had a pivotal role in early efforts at treatment and healing. She reported to Breuer a method of her own design that brought her relief and called it chimney sweeping. It was a state of autosuggestion or self hypnosis in which she would review events of the day. Breuer soon found that letting her report those events to him would bring further relief, a cleansing of sorts that Breuer enhanced with hypnotism and then called the cathartic method. The method brought temporary or short term relief and had to be repeated often. Breuer and Freud used the technique and both were disappointed with its limited ability to provide relief but no lasting cure. Some tension began to develop between them when Freud noted that the female patients seemed to be getting better as a means of expressing gratitude to their doctors for their attention. What supported this strongly was the fact that relapses occurred soon after either of them failed to attend to a patient. At this time, the early 1880's, Freud had no conception yet of transference or oedipal attachment and his explanation ended at the point of the patient rewarding the doctor both with improvement and an affectionate attachment. The latter soon created a storm of anxious concern for Breuer with Anna O.

A mutually affectionate attachment, not acted out, had been developing between Anna O and Breuer. His wife grew weary of listening to him speak of his work and became ever more jealous, not simply because of his attention to his work but certainly also because Anna was a young beauty with a charming personality. Breuer decided to abruptly end the treatment, with Anna O. She was at that time considerably improved but within the same day she developed severe symptoms again, one of which was pseuodcyesis (hysterical pregnancy). Breuer, overwhelmed by both conscious and unconscious awareness of the implications for his marriage left Vienna with his wife the very next day for a second honeymoon. Regrettably Anna O was left in a lurch and deteriorated quickly. Interestingly, Freud's wife Martha and Anna O were friends, making it likely that Freud was learning things about Anna O not disclosed during treatment.

In time the oedipal meaning behind Anna O's attachment to Breuer would come to Freud, but not for many more years. Aside from the limited rewards in patient improvement, Freud was deeply concerned at this time with his limited ability to hypnotize. He did not regard himself as good at hypnotism and could not hypnotize some patients at all. He experimented with ways to improve his technique such as insisting that his patients would recall key things about their symptoms during hypnosis. He also used pressure by hand on the patients' foreheads, but again with little result. He was convinced for a long time that if only he could put the patients into a deep enough hypnosis he would then obtain the data he needed to understand their disorders enough to be able to help them more. In time he abandoned this belief and came to regard hypnotism as a tool of limited use with the neuroses. On the way to this view of hypnosis he also tried other tools of his time such as electrotherapy, massage and baths but none of his efforts produced more improvement than the efforts of others at that time.

Freud began to notice, in small steps, that the more he quietly listened to his patients, the more narrative he obtained from them. There were subtle hints coming to him, and when some of them failed to be subtle, he learned a valuable lesson. In at least one case a female told him in so many words to shut up and let her continue with her story. The sum of all such happenings led him to realize that urging his patients or directly questioning them was of little use. He came to realize that an attitude of permissive, non-intrusive and non-judgmental listening produced far more data than hypnosis. He called this method free association, meaning that a patient was asked to report whatever came to mind or feeling, freely and without censorship. He developed and refined this method into the early 1890's. His method came to be called the talking cure, as expression created not by Freud, but by Anna O.

Although he now had a better method for securing data, he was slow to find its meanings. It was obvious to him that the more he worked with any one patient, the further back in that patient's life the narrative would take him. He had intuitions that causal events, though not yet discerned by him, were to be found in the earliest years of life, in childhood, by which he meant the first five years of life. When he began to see some of the meanings in the data, a number of difficulties arose that gave him pause but did not deter him. The data were suggesting sexual etiology in the neuroses. He was not prepared for such findings, first because he had no such expectation and no preconception as to where the data were leading him. In addition, his wish to communicate such findings would be counter to the Zeitgeist both among his colleagues and elsewhere. Regrettably this eventually led to a break with Breuer who could not deal with the idea of sexual etiology. However, in all the years that followed Freud cited Breuer as the originator of psychoanalysis because of his creation of the cathartic method, as his elaboration of Anna O's chimney sweeping came to be called.

Freud was certainly becoming something of a psychologist at this point but he still searched for purely medical causes. He investigated the prospect of toxins causing hysteria and the obsessional disorder but found nothing. Similarly he inquired into the role of genetics and found nothing. At one point he was sure that syphilitic infection in adults could result in a tendency to neurosis in their children, but further investigation led him to regard this line of thinking as untenable.

At this point Freud was still dominated by Charcot's ideas on traumas as basic causal factors in neurosis. This would mean, for example, that a disorder could arise as a result of the death of a loved one, financial ruin, divorce and so on. That is, strong enough stressful events were thought to be sufficient to drive the creation of symptoms of a disorder. The method of treatment at this time, the cathartic method, was also referred to as abreaction, meaning that if the patient could consciously re-experience the blocked affect or emotional charge of the original trauma then relief would follow, hence the term catharsis, which is Greek for cleansing or purifying. There were a number of problems with this position. Why was it that no amount of cathartic treatment would lead to permanent relief? What was it that was renewing the symptoms time after time? Most importantly, for Freud, why was it that cathartic treatment led to narrative on earlier and earlier life experiences and traumas?

Before fully parting from the trauma hypothesis Freud was initially convinced that he had found an answer. Many of his patients reported episodes of seduction in early childhood and many of these seemed to be reliable reports. If such seductions were behind every instance of illness then Freud would have reason to believe that he had found an original trauma and had succeeded in finally making sense of the data he was obtaining. It was quite a blow to him to learn that his hypothesis was not correct and it took him quite some time to recover himself from his disillusionment. He was in the very interesting and difficult position where much of his data suggested something that was not true. In releasing his attachment to the trauma theory he opened to a new formulation that would stand the test of time. He used his gift for letting his intuitive feelings tell him what the data *really* said and found a larger concept with which to account for his data. Here is what Freud had to say of this:

> "Under the influence of the technical procedure which I used at that time, the majority of my patients reproduced from their childhood scenes in which they were sexually seduced by some grow-up person. With female patients the part of seducer was almost always assigned to their father. I believed these stories, and consequently supposed that I had discovered the roots of the subsequent neurosis in these experiences of sexual seduction in childhood. My confidence was strengthened by a few cases in which relations of this kind with a father, uncle, or older brother had continued up to an age at which memory was to be trusted. If the reader feels inclined to shake his head at my credulity, I cannot altogether blame him, though I may plead that this was at a time when I was intentionally keeping my critical faculty in abeyance so as to preserve an unprejudiced and receptive attitude towards the many novelties which were coming to my notice very day. When, however, I was at last obliged to recognize that these scenes of seduction had never taken place, and that they were only phantasies which my patients had made up or which I myself had perhaps forced upon them, I was for some time completely at a loss. My confidence alike in my technique and in its results suffered a severe blow; it could not be disputed that I had arrived at these scenes by a technical method which I considered correct, and their subject-matter was unquestionably related to the symptoms from which my investigation had started. When I had pulled myself together, I was able to draw the right conclusions from my discovery: namely, that the neurotic symptoms were not related directly to actual events but to phantasies embodying wishes, and that as far as the neurosis was concerned, psychical reality was of more importance than material reality." (Freud, 2001, Vol XX, 33-34)

The last line of this passage expresses Freud's emergence as a psychologist, rather than only a neurologist treating emotional problems. It also expresses a major innovation in psychological thinking, that the way a person perceives or emotionally interprets what is happening is more important clinically than what is coming externally to the person. This is a relativistic idea and was formulated before Einstein's work on relativity was either published or generally known in some form to the public.[4] This line of thinking, when combined with his data taking him further and further back in a patient's life, led to some new concepts on pathology as well as on treatment.

The earlier idea of traumatic etiology was subsumed by the concepts of fixation and defense. Freud saw that pathology resulted from a developmental arrest, or fixation, of parts of the personality in childhood. The general idea of trauma entered as the child being presented with stresses beyond its young and emerging capacities to adapt. What had to be achieved was not abreaction but a lifting of defenses so that the once blocked drives could become conscious and resume the growth or maturation intended for them by nature from the outset. The role of a defense, as noted earlier, was to enable the unstressed parts of the personality to continue to grow as well as to spare the child the unmanageable pain of consciously experiencing what it could not deal with. At first Freud understood repression as a defense and used that word for defenses in general. With further research, especially into the obsessional disorder, he came to see that many more forms of defense existed such as reaction formation, rationalizing, undoing, projection (mostly in the case of paranoia), displacement, denial, dedifferentiation (in the case of psychosis) and so on.

Freud's divining these ideas from the patient's free associations led to the treatment idea of lifting the patient's defenses through a slow but accelerating use of interpretations. He often referred to the work of analysis as being a form of re-education but it was more a matter of building ego strength by gradually informing the patient's consciousness of the meaning of his or her emotional experiences. Healing and growth were achieved by the work of analysis to lift defenses that blocked drives from maturing. Within this model, symptoms resulted from the need of the blocked drives to discharge their energy. A healthy discharge, intended biologically as an adaptive behavior and tending toward growth, was not possible in the defended state, and the biological need to maintain homeostasis took place by alternate means of discharge resulting in symptoms, such as anxiety, depression, phobias, conversions (body expressions, such as paralysis), or pathological emotional states and so on.

Freud recognized that some maladies ought to be treated via hypnosis or catharsis, a position now evident in such things as PTSD. These symptom oriented methods were regarded as appropriate for maladies not

---

[4] The present discussion is referred to the late 1880's and early 1890's. Einstein published his work on special relativity in 1905. Freud and Einstein met at Freud's son's home in 1926, exchanged open letters on war in 1932 and personal letters in 1936.

rooted in childhood fixation, these being the neuroses and psychoses. He often summarized the goal of psychoanalysis as being to make the unconscious conscious, for the reasons given. This points to a fundamental difference between the earlier, symptom oriented methods and analysis. While both look to provide relief by liberating what is unconscious – abreaction versus lifting of defenses – there are differences in context. Where abreaction is appropriate there is no significant issue of childhood developmental arrest but rather the restoration of a more functional state of the personality. With the neuroses, the issue is not restoration but the enabling of healing and growth, the latter failing to take place in childhood.

Freud was beginning to see some of the unconscious dynamics at work in the neurotic state. The above ideas clearly imply the existence of an unconscious conflict. In its early formulation this was seen as one between drives (id derivatives) and the safety or well being of the patient. One part of the personality was trying to come into expression while another part regarded such expression as dangerous, giving rise to a blocking agent termed a defense. Within this model the perception of danger, like the drive itself, is unconscious and the defense arises spontaneously, much along the lines of a reflex, to protect the child. For the child, the ultimate issue is its need to safeguard the parental love that preserves and promotes its life. An unconscious part of the personality perceives that expression of the given drives would be objectionable to the child's parents and leads to another unconscious part, reflex wise, creating a defense to block it. The danger here relates to the prospect of losing parental love and Freud eventually used this to define guilt as fear of loss of love. The goal of treatment was to promote healing and growth via interpretations that enabled the conscious personality to see that there were unconscious parts of it – the personality – working against its adaptation and well being. The healing aspect refers to the lifting or dissolving of defenses as the patient is made to see them and their maladaptive work. The growth aspect results from the once blocked id derivatives becoming free to resume the unfolding that was arrested by the defenses in childhood. Freud used the reflex analogy to draw attention to the fact that defenses, like the drives they work against, arise on their own and are not summoned forward by either an act of will or by consciousness; both arising from unconscious sources, the latter depending upon powers of unconscious perception that make their creation necessary for the child's survival and continued growth.

Over time Freud crystallized these formulations into the idea that a neurosis is an ego/id conflict, where unconscious parts of the ego erect defenses to block id drives perceived as dangerous. The idea of the superego eventually entered as that part of the psyche that generated guilt if the ego considered fulfilling dangerous drives; the superego was also a source of self esteem in the opposite case of compliance where certain drives or behaviors were perceived as 'good' and could be expressed. Thus, the superego repeated from within the psyche the once external role of the parents to punish (guilt) versus reward (self esteem or endorsement). Freud used these terms to define depression and mania as outcomes of an ego/superego conflict and to define a psychosis as an ego reality conflict. More on these models of pathology will follow later, however, it should be said now that these formulas are more than explanatory models for psychopathology because they indicate where conflict is located and hence identify elements of treatment. In a sense they indicate what an interpretation ought to target and how to present it.

Freud's initial work with hysterics and obsessionals led to the postulating of stages of psychosexual development as fixation points that characterized the disorders. The least among the neuroses in severity, hysteria, corresponds to fixation in the third such stage, the genital stage, sometimes referred to as the phallic stage. He regarded this stage as characterized by a coming together of prior sexual components, under genital primacy, that until this time acted mostly independently of one another. He also regarded this coming together as ushering in the Oedipus complex, in which a child develops a possessive attachment to its opposite sex parent with feelings of hostile rivalry directed at its same sex parent. The phrase phallic stage is used to emphasize the Oedipus complex as part of the genital stage. The phrase genital primacy means that the component instincts now act together, synergistically, to lead to genital excitement that builds to orgasm regardless of how the components may have initially been stimulated.

He felt that the use of repression and of fantasies formed the major defenses at this point. The root conflict in the oedipal longing is fear of loss of love from and punishment by the same sex parent. This event, a milestone in the development of human love, occurs around age three and lasts about one to one and a half years. It is a milestone in love because it is the first time that a human being feels other directed love for someone rather than only love dependent on need gratification. The word hysteria is derived from the Greek υστερα (hystera), meaning womb because the disorder was observed in antiquity mostly in women and hence came to be associated with their anatomy. Freud took this etymology to reflect a knowing in the ancients of a connection between aspects of sexual conflict and hysteria. Further research established that the disorder occurs with comparable frequency in males and that the use of a stereotypy (Krohn,

1978) characterizes it in both genders, the stereotypy having some connection with hysterical fantasies. Some common stereotypies are the femme fatale in the female and the mover and shaker in both genders. They are, in part, compensations for the literal impossibility of actually winning the oedipal competition because the stereotype is perceived as being an actual role in life that the child can carry out, creating some sense of compensatory success for the inevitable oedipal defeat.

There is more than fear of loss of love of the same sex parent in the child's oedipal anxieties. In the case of the male the child fears castration because he understands, at some unconscious level, that this will remove his ability to compete with the father for the mother, making him unable to take his place with her. It would also be a grave narcissistic injury. In the case of the female the dreaded punishment is loss of the ability to bear children, sometimes referred to evisceration anxiety – the parallel to castration anxiety – in which the child unconsciously fears the mother tearing out her reproductive system. Here also there is a narcissistic injury of profound concern. It is worth noting here that both anxieties occur with frequency in the world's mythologies and both form organizing themes in much of the world's literature and art.

Although Freud distinguished anxiety hysteria from conversion hysteria, the underlying dynamics are the same. Aside from anxiety as a diagnostic sign of the first form, emotional flooding was often also diagnostic, as suggested by the convention of referring to people in overly emotional states as being hysterical. With conversion hysteria, the unconscious conflict is expressed in abnormal body states such as hysterical blindness, paralysis, choking or even false pregnancy (pseudocyesis) in which the patient's unconscious creates some or all of the physical signs of pregnancy, including breaking of water, labor pains, pelvic dilation and a delivery, not of a child, but of fluid. The fact that unconscious fantasies found in conversion hysteria defined the form of the conversion symptoms led him to regard a conversion symptom as expressing a specific meaning. In the well known case of Dora Freud traced her psychogenic cough to a conflict between oedipal fantasies of fellatio with her lover and her oedipal guilt feelings that would equate the lover with her father. In a number of hysterics suffering with contractures that resulted in sexually suggestive positioning, the unconscious fantasies were likewise traced to conflicted longings for incest with the father and guilt feelings. He found that in general conversion symptoms have a meaning related to unconscious fantasies but not every somatic symptom of emotional origin does. For example, blocked rage can lead to hypertension but the symptom expresses no meaning trying to reach consciousness, rather it expresses the over-mobilization caused by the ongoing attempt of the rage to come into conscious expression and discharge.

The therapeutic goal with hysteria is the use of interpretations to lift the patient's repressions, as well as other secondary defenses, so as to slowly build the ego strength required for the patient to see the underlying oedipal conflict and the unconscious fantasies associated with it. The point is to go from cognitive understanding to emotionally re-experiencing the oedipal attachment in consciousness, the latter achieving resolution far more than the former. When Freud first did this he expected cognitive understanding to lead to healing and growth more quickly than actually happened. This led him to the concept of resistance which has some relatedness to his comments on defenses being reflex like. A reflex is a physiological given that takes place immediately and, initially, out of awareness in response to certain stimuli, giving it the property of autonomy. It is difficult to create or extinguish a reflex although behaviorists have made considerable progress in this area. Although Freud used the reflex analogy to draw attention to the autonomy and regularity with which a defense works, the idea of resistance is more related to the idea of inertia in physics, a concept he was well aware of. The basic idea is that any material system will tend to function as it has until the present moment unless it experiences an intervention that alters its progression. Resistance refers to the inertial tendency of defenses to continue to function after childhood is over as they did within childhood. This leads to the treatment issue of how to deal with resistance.

The intervention of choice is, of course, the interpretation of the patient's narrative, symptoms and dreams. If patient and analyst are well enough matched, this usually leads to healing and growth, but not always. Freud had two ways of dealing with resistance in order to accelerate therapeutic progress in analysis. He felt that it was important for patients to confront their anxieties, to do what was important to them even though it resulted in unwelcome feelings. This procedure is now more often called force functioning, sometimes powering through, and it accelerates the therapeutic process because doing what is wanted in the presence of negative, opposing feelings tends to erode defenses more quickly than otherwise. His second policy, with a patient who was overly resistant, was to give a deadline for the end of the analysis. He did this in the famous case of the Wolf Man and it worked. This was a case that began as anxiety hysteria and then changed into an obsessional disorder; it is referred to as the Wolf Man case because the patient had an anxiety dream of six or seven white wolves perched on a walnut tree outside his bedroom window, the dream playing a major role in his analysis.

Somewhat related to resistance was the issue of how to accelerate the therapeutic process. Freud noted how patients would tend to act out infantile wishes in their sessions in the hope of getting him to fulfil them. That this is a transference issue will be treated in Chapter 6. Freud understood intuitively that mending a neurosis involved growing up and that no gain could result from satisfying said infantile wishes. At the same time he saw that frustrating those wishes would stress the patient's defenses and accelerate their demise. A proof of sorts of this arose in practice when hysterics would flood more as their defenses failed and the necessary experience of once blocked drives becoming conscious occurred.

Much of the foregoing on hysteria and the genital stage illustrates how the ego, id, superego model arose from studying psychopathology. It identifies where conflict is located and indicates elements of treatment. In summary form an hysteric is developmentally arrested in the genital stage with id derived oedipal strivings that are opposed dominantly by the ego defense of repression. Guilt over such strivings is directed at the same sex parent and is superego generated. This assumes that the given person has no significant fixations in earlier stages. The event that enables the Oedipus complex is the coming together or prior id component instincts that now work in collaboration in relation to a more mature ego. The use of a stereotypy is another ego defense used to manage the perception of the oedipal attachment as being dangerous by allowing the person to seek success in the stereotyped area. Fantasies are also used defensively by the ego in conjunction with the id, this being a primary process event to be discussed later. The symptoms in hysteria, whether anxiety or conversion hysteria, are the result of the ego regulating discharge of id tendencies. The ego, being unable to satisfy the original tendencies because of superego and reality constraints, establishes other, associatively related means of discharge, these being symptoms because they are not the discharge of id energy intended by nature in the healthy state. This applies to all symptoms and not just those of hysteria.

Treatment proceeds by using interpretations to inform the patient's conscious ego of unconscious repressions directed at id strivings. Over time this builds the ego strength to move the patient from what is initially mostly cognitive understanding to the ability to also experience in awareness once again the id strivings (emotionally charged strivings) blocked by repression, as well as by some other, supporting defenses, since childhood. With successful treatment the automatism of the defenses diminishes and with it resistance. Freud's chief way of dealing with resistance was to encourage, if not push, patients into force functioning where they pursue things of importance to them in the face of opposing feelings such as anxiety. This results in increased ego strength for reprocessing once blocked id drives as the lifting of defenses enables them to approach awareness. It also increases ego strength for dealing with superego driven guilt over the id drives.

Freud's work with patients' infantile demands, typically to be mothered, fathered or coddled, led to the formation of the idea of transference, to be treated later. At issue is that he found that frustrating such demands tended to erode defenses and promote growth in ego strength.

At various times, and depending on the patient's readiness, interpretations are offered to the conscious ego to create/increased awareness of oedipal longings (id), the use of defenses (ego) or the presence of guilt (superego). Interpretation of symptoms creates awareness of distorted means of emotional discharge – neurotic regulation of id strivings by the ego – eroding ego defenses and, in the case of successful treatment, leading to emotionally corrective experiences in which discharge takes place more as intended by nature for the healthy state.

Freud's work with obsessionals led to the formulation of a psychosexual stage before the genital one, the anal stage. He did not regard the genital stage as supplanting the anal but rather as both emerging from it and subsuming it within cumulative development. Most of the component instincts Freud regarded as coming together in genital fusion arise in the anal stage, especially the early part, often referred to as the anal sadistic stage. Some such components are sadism, an early and not yet mature form of mastery, epistemophilia, a knowledge seeking instinct and scoptophilia, an instinct for looking. Another component instinct, carried over from the earlier oral stage, is that of contrectation, an instinct for touching, necessary to support the rooting reflex and maternal contact immediately after birth.

A systemic outcome of the anal stage is the emergence of the secondary process, which has two aspects. The affective part of this process is in the child learning to use its emerging aggression to forego instant satisfactions in favor of eventual, and greater ones, this being a form of frustration tolerance. This is often called the reality principle and is a special case of what happens generally in the anal stage where powerful aggressive instincts emerge for the first time, destined in the state of health to unfold into adaptive powers of mastery; the specific power of mastery cited here is over the self in the acquisition of frustration tolerance. Freud often referred to the general maturational goal of the aggressive instincts as the creation of reality modifying powers. The other major aspect of the secondary process, often called reality sense, is a cognitive outcome of the anal stage. Within the anal stage the child becomes increasingly able to distinguish between and among objects that differ in reality, the child's earlier form of knowing being based on recognizing groups of things.

The anal stage is so named because the emergence of aggressive powers and reality testing powers (adaptive use of the reality sense) occurs as the child acquires erotic sensations in the anal area, this being attended by central nervous system growth that supports the sensations. Three things are noteworthy of this stage: the affective or instinctual event of aggressive powers coming forward, the cognitive event of reality sense and reality testing appearing and the affective event of anal eroticism arising. Developmental arrest in this stage is associated with the obsessional disorder. This can arise in two ways or as a mix of the two. If the child experiences overly strong anxiety and stress during its oedipal attachment in the genital stage, it will, in whole or in part, abandon its oedipal strivings and regress back to the prior stage, the anal stage, where it had fared better and could sustain the presenting stresses with more success, but at the cost of arrest that results in neurotic limitations, to be noted. The other way it can occur is with the presentation too much stress in the anal stage itself, making the advance to the genital stage both limited and precarious, meaning that some advance into the genital stage takes place but is broken off by stress that makes a regression back to the anal stage necessary.

The three things noted above of the anal stage identify the characteristics of the obsessional disorder. As repression is a defining defense for hysteria, a reaction formation is a defining defense for the obsessional. Whether driven by excessive oedipal stress such as castration anxiety or by excessive stress within the anal stage itself, or both, the outcome for the child consists of strong rage reactions, these being an unrehearsed and automatic aggressive reaction to the presenting stresses. The child is made by nature to know inwardly that it must not allow its rage reactions to come into expression with its parents because such actions may put its survival at risk. This is a guilt reaction (fear of loss of love) that leads to the defining defense of a reaction formation in which the child unconsciously uses some of its aggression to bind the rest of it away from consciousness and from access to parts of the personality that have sufficient access to consciousness to be perceived as risky. Secondarily, some of the aggressive energy of the rage is used to express the opposite of what is blocked resulting in personality traits of exaggerated kindness, mercy, sympathy and the like, these being overcompensations that cloak the hate blocked by the reaction formation.

Since the reaction formed is laid down early in life subsequent emotional development takes place within the context of its inhibiting/blocking presence. This implies that the blocking action of the defense tends to also block any emotion that has sufficient relatedness to aggression. The outcome, within the disorder, is that obsessionals tend to have weak contact with their feelings and emotions in large parts of their personalities. The rigidity of the defense is seen in a general rigidity of personality that welcomes sameness and avoids nuance or change. Their observable interactions overemphasize thinking and underemphasize feeling. Indeed, it is a standing quip that one can diagnose an obsessional by asking how he or she feels about something and when the replies are thoughts rather than feelings, there is a telltale sign of an obsessional. The analogous quip with an hysteric is to ask what he or she thinks of something and to then observe a reply rich in emotion and feelings. The general rigidity and favoring of sameness is seen in the systematic way obsessionals adapt. The system evolves from the anal stage forward and becomes a complex set of responses to cues that avoids or minimizes aggressive expression or self experience.

Freud noted that certain character traits tend to cluster in an obsessional, such as chronic over-concern with time, orderliness, parsimony and money. He traced this to the simultaneity of toilet training and the emergence of secondary process abilities, the connecting link being that toilet training involves issues of time, order and mastery. These character traits together with the presence of the obsessional system led Freud to make a number of comments about them. He often referred to the illness as that remarkable disorder, having in mind how surprising it is that a person can have such a divide between thinking and feeling and yet not be psychotic. He also often referred to it as that crazy disorder when he observed how convoluted, complex and removed from reality obsessions can become. The case of the Rat Man and the complexity of how he planned to pay a debt, too long to detail here, is one such example. Freud felt that this craziness resulted from the secondary process cognitive aspect being utilized to avoid things ever more remote from the original dreaded object based on such things having weak cognitive likeness to the original. This is actually an example of primary process functioning in symptom formation and will be developed more carefully in chapter 5. Their emphasis on secondary process logic and their avoidance of feeling usually result in high cognitive intelligence and at best mediocre emotional intelligence in them. He was taken with the inner state of obessionals and the impact of the often enormous amount of rage their defenses work to contain. This led, inevitably, to reactive guilt which in turn led to considerable self hurtful behaviors that worked to dampen the guilt. So great was the rage and reactive guilt he observed that he often said that the amount of guilt seen in obsessionals would be appropriate in a mass murderer. Similarly, he was fond of saying that obsessionals are always finding new ways to punish themselves

Along more positive lines he referred to obsessionals as the true upholders of society. Two strains of thought led him to this. For one, when obsessionals function within their systems they are usually highly productive and efficient. For another, they tend to have overly strong moral standards as part of their guilt driven rigidity and to such a degree that Freud often said of them that they practiced a private religion, this being their system. The joint effect of their working within their obsessional systems with high ethical standards led him to refer to them as the true upholders of society. No doubt it was also a self reference because he self diagnosed as one of them.

Episodic depression is usually found in the obsessional because the central defense or reaction formation can fail under sufficient stress and also when collateral defenses prove insufficient. The outcome is that some of the once blocked rage can begin to reach parts of the waking personality or parts that have access to it. This recreates the original feeling of being overwhelmed in the anal stage and leads to fresh secondary defensive maneuvers to once again keep the rage away from awareness and whatever can link with it. The main maneuver is an alliance with unconscious guilt, ever strong in the obsessional, that leads to some of the now free aggression turning upon the self and driving depressive symptoms. This is not tantamount to a depressive disorder but is rather a depressive episode.

Neurotic versus healthy homosexual trends are part of the disorder. As noted the anal stage is so called because of the emergence of erotic anal sensations arising in it as a pregenital stage. That is, the subject has not yet evolved to the point where the distinction between male and female is known in an emotional sense, this being an outcome of the next stage. The close proximity of the anus to the vagina results in strange and often comic theories of sex and birth in children that tend to continue into adult life. At the same time the fact that both genders have an anus leads to further limited ability to yet distinguish the genders. This, coupled with the natural pleasure of anal sensations tends to lead to pregenital homosexual trends in the obsessional that are healthy at the time of their emergence but sometimes unhealthy when continued into adult life. Neurotic versus healthy homosexual trends are determined by both the degree of successful advance into the genital stage and the degree of anal fixation.

Freud saw the anal sadistic stage as ushering in many component instincts whose expression defined the perversions. Sadism, the taking of pleasure in inflicting pain is a prime example. Coprophilia, necrophilia and exhibitionism are others. Freud's ability to use his feelings to gather knowledge is apparent in his treatment of the perversions. The first order of business was to define what a perversion is and for this he distinguished between the aim and the object of an instinct. With sexuality the aim is pleasure and the object is properly a person. If the aim becomes inappropriate such as looking to achieve domination and control or if the object is inappropriate such as in bestiality, the resulting behavior is said to be perverse. In formula form a perversion is the expression of an instinct in which either the aim or object or both of the instinct is inappropriate. Freud was well aware that people, including himself before his research, tended to group neurotics and perverts into the same class, leading him to study their differences more closely. The result of his study was the formula that perversions are the opposite of neuroses because in the former instincts are freely acted out or expressed but in the latter they are opposed by defenses. In the former the ego sees no danger, this including superego pressure or guilt, in the given instinct(s) being allowed the pursuit of their satisfaction, but in the latter there is perceived danger, including guilt, in giving certain instincts free rein and hence they are blocked or thwarted by defenses.

Treatment of the obsessional has two central goals. The first is to use interpretations to inform the ego of the conflict between id derived rage, which drives guilt, and the ego itself whose task is to manage the rage, but away from consciousness. The whole point of the disorder is to keep blocked rage away from or even near access to the waking personality, a thing that can only result in the usual symptoms of obsessing, compulsing, anxiety and episodic depression. The second goal arises from the fact that the great amount of rage which makes a reaction formation necessary results in a general emotional rigidity, this making it necessary, as is often said, to work to make the obsessional more human. Both goals rely on the use of interpretations to both inform and to move the personality toward more lability, usually a long term and slow process.

The fixation point for the obsessional is early enough for the resulting ego capacities to be quite short of what life needs for successful adaptation. When this is coupled with the fact that the obsessional is still in a state where he or she is waiting either for the relief of the stresses driving the disorder and/or for the life creating emotional cues needed for healing and growth, then it becomes clear that dependency is another significant treatment issue. The goal of using interpretations to lift defenses and resolve the rage driven ego/id conflict also includes work to increase ego strength. Freud and his following rely on encouraging the patient to confront his or her anxieties. As noted earlier, this is usually called force functioning, where the patient is urged to pursue things either of necessity or interest in the presence of opposing feelings. The idea is partly to desensitize the person but it is more to accelerate the breakdown of defenses that maintain the neurotic state.

A corollary to the obsessional's comparatively low ego strength is the presence of infantile coping mechanisms, yet to be outgrown.[5] Chief among them is magical thinking where a person believes that his or her thoughts influence the course of reality. It is a companion to the superstitious trends and animism seen in obsessionals where the latter refers to the belief that inanimate objects are alive or have some powers not properly found in them but only in living things. A stone or a tree or even a car that feels and can think are common examples in children, as seen in folklore.

In terms of Freud's structured model, the therapeutic task includes promoting sublimations of the blocked rage, an ego/id task, and downgrading unconscious guilt, an ego/superego task. Promoting sublimations leads both to more lability as well as to more reality oriented, useful powers of adaptation – the once blocked rage becomes an energy source for the generation of such powers. The fact that such work leads to a better life can only be opposed by unconscious guilt and this relates the first task to the second. When successful the second task also leads to increases in self esteem. The central target of interpretive work is to undo the reaction formation but it also includes undoing other supporting defenses often found in the obsessional such as denial, undoing, repression and rationalization. From Freud's time forward this has been a slow and laborious process because the ego holds tightly to its dread of being overwhelmed, even annihilated, by the liberation of the blocked id rage.

The points of developmental arrest can cover more than the anal stage, and in any one case, can fall anywhere from the early oral stage to the late genital stage; In general, the arrest points for any neurosis lie in the interval from the late oral stage to the late genital stage. Since the arrest

---

[5] A coping mechanism is a means of dealing with adaptive challenges that brings comfort without denying the negative aspects of the challenge; procrastination is an example. This is to be distinguished from a defense mechanism where the quest for comfort is also present but the goal is to keep the negative aspects, the underlying pathology, away from awareness.

points can be multiple, that is falling in different stages, it follows that a person can have both obsessional and hysterical configurations at the same time. The 'pure' hysterical and obsessional descriptions given here can only be approximated to in reality, the former where there is genital fixation and little of any other kind, and the latter where there is anal fixation and little else. To say that someone is hysterical means that the major neurotic trend in the person is hysterical even though there are lesser obsessional trends, and similarly for typing someone as obsessional.

Freud's theory of psychosexual stages does not end with the genital stage ,the stages of as latency and puberty coming next. However, he found that there is little, if any possibility, of psychological illness being created after the genital stage, a time that he felt corresponded to about age five, most of the time. He felt that the lifelong structure of the personality was in something of a final basic form at the end of the genital stage, the concept being similar to how the frame of a building defines how the rest of it is filled in. The concept applies to both health and illness with the proviso that the basic structure, in the case of illness, can often be altered with suitable psychotherapy.

These comments are offered here because the amount of decrease in differentiation in going backwards from the genital to the anal stage is small when compared to that in going from the anal to the oral. They are also offered here because the narrative is building to the use of the primary process, an outcome of the oral stage, to describe many aspects of healing and growth. In addition the oral stage is set apart by certain distinguishing features, to be developed now.

At the moment of birth a neonate is equipped with a very basic survival tool, the rooting reflex. It inclines a neonate to respond to the touch of anything that is soft, warm and round with a reflex search for a nipple for suckling. The reflex is quite indiscriminate, responding to the presentation of a shoulder, an upper arm or even an abdomen in the same way. This is noteworthy because being indiscriminate, that is, having low powers of differentiated perception, characterizes the primary process. A second example of weak differentiation is the smiling response.[6] At the average age of three months an infant will respond to the presentation of any moving object that has features resembling a forehead, eyes and nose with a smile, provided that it is presented face forward and not in profile. The lack of differentiation in the response is seen in the fact that even a mask so configured will elicit a smile. (Spitz) Within the oral stage the

---

[6] References to the smiling response, here and subsequently, are due to Spitz, (Spitz, 1965)

primary process matures as the baby comes to recognize more object types. The relevance, to be developed fully later in chapter 5 is that the primary process perceives not objects but the classes to which they belong, the smiling response being a good example of this.

The object of major concern in the oral stage is, of course, the mother. The mother's offering of life creating love gives the infant cues that invite its personality forward. When the love is consistent and reliable enough the infant's personality develops healthily. However, when this is not the case two forms of pathology can arise, one being schizophrenia and the other depressive psychosis.[7] The fact that developmental arrest in this stage can result in two different maladies sets it apart from both the anal and genital stages where only one broad type of malady can result, this being the obsessional in the anal stage and the hysteric in the genital stage. It is also set apart by its being the first stage, implying that all subsequent healthy unfolding depends upon its healthy unfolding.

Freud was not fond of working with psychotics because he felt that they usually have too little capacity to form a transference, this being an outcome of the strong narcissism found in psychoses. However, he did feel that work with psychotics could be of value for research into the personality in general because their early points of developmental arrest implied that early psychic systems or parts could be observed directly before they differentiated or unfolded into higher order systems. The yield, he argued, would be insight into early structure and form, mostly of the ego. With this in mind, he made contributions to their understanding. In the case of schizophrenia, where developmental arrest is caused by deficient mothering in the early oral stage, he described the outcome as an internal catastrophe. The word schizophrenia is from the Greek words σχιζειν (schizein), meaning to split, cleave or separate and φρην (phren), meaning soul, mind or heart. In its roots schizophrenia is about fragmentation of personality, a key sign of the disorder. Hallucinations, in which thoughts and inner images are taken to be sensory perceptions outside the self is an example. Likewise delusions in which reality is grossly misinterpreted are also an example. The use of language in schizophrenia, often called word salad, also illustrates the characteristic fragmentation. The term word salad refers to the jumbled and nonsensical form of verbal responses from schizophrenics, reminiscent of how the various parts of a salad become randomly tossed together.

---

[7] There are also biological causes of the psychoses, but they are outside the present concerns.

The fragmentation of personality is clear in the above examples, and though it is entirely nonsensical, the schizophrenic use of language can be shown to make sense at another level by reference to how the primary process enters in its formation. Freud felt that dominance of primary process functioning characterizes the psychoses, and more generally, that such functioning is seen in all forms of pathology to varying degrees .Making sense of the schizophrenic use of language will be revisited at the end of Chapter 4 which presents material on the primary process.

Paranoia is usually considered to be a subtype of schizophrenia. Without going into the relation of blocked homosexuality and castration anxiety to its genesis, the idea of fragmentation of personality is seen here in a nearly transparent way. Paranoids are said to have unshakeable beliefs, an aspect of their delusional defenses. Here the person's reality testing fails to connect with perceptions of the emotional meanings of things and the perceptions are then reworked as verifications of the delusional system. The fragmentation here is evident in the wide separation between perception and reality testing. The treatment goal here, to restore reality testing, almost always fails because of the astonishing degree of rigidity in the paranoid as well as the patient's efforts to work the therapist into his or her delusional system.

With healthy mothering the various parts of the infant's personality emerge and begin a first integration. In the case of schizophrenia, either certain parts fail to come forward or, if they do, they fail to integrate. It is possible for this to be so severe that the disorder begins in childhood in which case it is usually referred to as autism, a disorder that can be fatal. However, what usually happens is that the personality achieves a fragile level of realization in the oral stage that supports some progress into the anal and genital stages, this collapsing usually during puberty under the stress of new and strong sexual and aggressive drives emerging. The collapse, or decompensation, can occur after adolescence also, and in all cases what tentative structures were achieved in ego, id and superego formation are undone in part, this being dedifferentiation; this is what Freud labelled an internal catastrophe. It is usually attended by bizarre symptoms such as delusions and hallucinations, the language symptom being a more chronic rather than acute symptom. Organismic panic is a major symptom in the acute state, a phrase used to describe the patient's inner but helpless awareness of the fragmentation, or breaking apart, of his or her personality. It is common for patients in this state to compensate with delusions of being a messianic or all powerful figure, the delusion reflecting the wish to have the strength or power to not break into pieces but to remain as one. Similarly they may hallucinate the appearance of such figures or their voices, the latter being more frequent.

Treatment of schizophrenia focuses on undoing the developmental arrests in the oral stage, a nontrivial task because the unfolding of the personality in the later stages depends upon enough unfolding in the earlier oral stage and because there is limited capacity to work with a psychoanalyst in the first place. As noted, Freud felt that treatment prospects for psychotics were poor or nonexistent because of their difficulty in forming a transference. The issue for Freud was that psychoanalysis uses the transference to recreate the original stresses that drove the formation of a neurosis so as to make them observable to both patient and analyst. This is followed by deliberate frustration of the patient's transference of those stresses and associated wishes and hence, if a patient cannot transfer then that patient cannot be treated, this being the heart of Freud's objection. However, work by his later following found other means for treating schizophrenia, based mostly on an inversion of Freud's objection. The later following found that offering the patient satisfaction of its frustrated infantile needs for mothering often results in healing and growth, a thing simply untrue of work with neurotics. The focus of the healing and growth for a schizophrenic is the ego, just budding at the time of birth. The preponderance of ego dysfunction in psychosis inclined Freud to call the psychoses a study in infantile ego development, and the work of his following substantiates his premise. His corresponding phrase for the neuroses is that they are studies in infantile sexuality because of the work to unblock id drives, or in the case of the perversions, to manage them.

A major developmental outcome of the oral stage is the laying down of the primary process. Although Freud regarded it as a law of the id, it is also a lower ego function as will be explained later. The laying down of the primary process occurs in the early oral stage where developmental failure can lead to schizophrenia as well as in the latter part of the oral stage where such failure can lead to depressive psychosis.[8] In the early oral stage the mother's role is mostly on inviting the child's personality forward with her love and presence. At this time the infant is still in a highly undifferentiated state so that the infant and the mother are not yet experienced or seen as distinct but rather as part of a monad. As development advances into the latter oral stage, the infant's ability to distinguish between self and mother emerges, a prerequisite for internalization of the mother. When such internalization fails or is not

---

[8] Freud regarded the primary process as present in elementary form at birth.

complete enough depressive psychosis can result. Freud's work on melancholia helps to make sense of this, In comparing mourning and melancholy or depression, Freud, building on the earlier work of Abraham, found striking parallels between the two with the single exception that mourning does not feature a diminished self esteem as occurs in depression and he took this as a key to understanding depression.

Within his model in both mourning and depression there is a loss but with the difference that in the former the loss of a person is real or objective and in the latter it is subjective, as in losing a person's love or high regard, failing to win endorsement of a needed person in work and so on. Freud felt that in depression the patient identifies with the lost object or person in order to keep it alive in some sense, and then turns his hate, reactive to the loss, upon that image. Since the hated image is now a part of the self, the rage is self directed, with the patient blaming himself for the loss, a familiar mechanism in creating depression. This results in the self loathing and self berating that connects with the cruel workings of the superego against the ego in this case, the ego being blamed as it were. These ideas lift in a natural way into explaining depressive psychosis.

As the infant unfolds in the later oral stage it grows the ability to unconsciously distinguish the satisfying ('good') versus frustrating or hurtful ('bad') parts of the mother, this being an aspect of ongoing differentiation. The mother's life creating love invites the infant's personality forward with the infant identifying with it leading to the laying down of an image of this aspect of the mother, usually referred to as the good object.[9] Similarly, the frustrating aspects of the mother are internalized with the resulting image usually referred to as the bad object. With healthy development the bad object gives rise to growth of frustration tolerance. In healthy development these two images are destined to become integrated into a single representation of the mother. Any frustration with the mother leads to a guilt reaction in the infant in association with the bad object within; the infant then blaming itself for its pain. When the frustration or hurt is severe enough the guilty accusations of the emerging superego overwhelm the infant's capacity and the foundation for depressive psychosis results. This is similar to what happens with neurotic depression but with some key differences. The amount of ego structure present to deal with the frustration is far less in the infant than with precursors to neurosis, and the superego itself is in a very early stage of formation, both leading to profound underdevelopment of the personality as a whole.

---

[9] References to the good or bad object, splitting and merging, here and subsequently are due to the work of Melanie Klein (Klein, 1975)

When in the adult state the given person experiences enough frustration he will re-experience the raging of his superego against the bad object, again felt as overwhelming and leading to reactivation or intensification of his early defenses.

The break with reality that characterizes psychosis appears in a number of ways. In the acute state, when the inner sense of guilt and emptiness is massive, the patient may hallucinate that the mother (or mothering figure) is present, this being a defense that looks to put the source of the persecuting superego back outside where it came from, a defense by externalization. The inner feeling that the good mother is gone and that life is at risk often results in hallucinations of the end of the world, rich in apocalyptic imagery; delusions of being a savior also enter as in schizophrenia but here the role of the delusion is not to thwart fragmentation but to redeem the world, that is, undo the bad object and replace it with more of the good object. Another defense, triggered not only by depressive pain but also by the immense helplessness the patient feels is merging, where the patient's sense of a boundary between self and other diminishes or vanishes, enabling a perception or experience of the life and power of the other person as being in the self, an attempt to increase good object internalization.

Because the early and later oral stages overlap and unfold over a short amount of time it is common for a patient to present with both schizophrenic and depressive psychotic trends, a condition referred to as schizoaffective. As with schizophrenia the therapeutic outlook is poor but some progress can be made by the analyst taking on the role of the wished for good mother to build up ego strength.

The nosology presented may seem to divide pathology into neurosis versus psychosis. The boundary between them is not well defined and those who fall in this symptomatic region are called borderline patients. A major surface defining trait of a borderline is that under nominal conditions of stress the patient behaves neurotically but with sufficient levels of stress the patient behaves increasingly psychotically, a trait that makes sense of the term borderline. The defining inner structure, or defense, of a borderline is splitting, an outcome of the failure to achieve an adequate integration of the good and bad object representations, beginning with the mother. In practical terms this means that a borderline responds to the satisfying and frustrating aspects of a person as if they were two different people. The implied limitations in love are obvious as are the implied limitations in ego strength for their work life, this being usually limited to menial labor, with frequent job changes. Their defense of choice, merging, is expectable for a number of reasons. The infantile part of their ego unconsciously sees the other person as potentially being the good object that can ameliorate or undo splitting because the arrival of the good object would greatly diminish the bad object. At the same the higher ego strength of the merged with person is seen as a solution to their inner sense of limited capacity and helplessness before the challenges of life. The greater self esteem of the merged with person is also seen as a source of relief for their low self esteem and frequent episodes of depression common in borderlines; their neediness is reminiscent of depressives.

Psychoanalytic treatment is similar to that with psychotics although borderlines have a higher capacity for interpretive work and somewhat more ego strength. The need for the therapist to assume parental roles while building up ego strength is clear. Unfortunately, their low frustration tolerance and need to merge usually make borderlines difficult to work with and call for more compassion and commitment than otherwise.

This chapter has been mostly about how Freud's wish to understand the psychoneuroses drew him increasingly into psychology and away from a purely medical approach. It is true that given his interests and talents this was a natural outcome, but it is also true that the scientific means of his time could not support the biological approach he began with. The final part of this chapter has been about the oral stage and the disorders associated with it because those disorders, the psychoses, are dominated by primary process functioning, a point of convergence in this book. Nonetheless, there is a point in Freud's career that is regarded by many as the time of his full commitment to a purely psychological approach. This event is marked by his publication of a work in which he made his last effort to construct a biological model of the personality. It is also marked by the fact that having dropped the effort because if its infeasibility, it happened that many of his basic and most valuable psychological ideas were presented in first form in the work, to be detailed in the next chapter.

CHAPTER 3

FREUD'S "PROJECT"

In 1895 Freud enthusiastically set to work on a new manuscript. He gave it no name but over time it came to be called "Project for a Scientific Psychology." His goal was to investigate feasible relationships between psychology and brain anatomy. Shortly before this time, in 1888, the Spanish anatomist Santiago Ramón y Cajal published findings on neurons, including the roles of axons and dendrites. It drew attention from many quarters in Europe, including Freud's as a neurologist. Freud sensed many implications of the idea that neurons could communicate with one another and this motivated him to try to identify possible relationships between groups of neurons and specific behaviors and functions.

The German edition of his work was given the title Entwurf einer Psychologie which translates as Outline of a Psychology. The masculine noun Entwurf can translate as sketch, outline, draft, rough copy, design, model, project, plan or scheme and suggests that the German editors understood that Freud's work was both new and ambitious. The translators of the original German into English created the now standard title "Project for a Scientific Psychology," a title more suggestive of Freud's goal. He worked on the project in the latter part of 1895 and originally intended to arrive at some biological/psychological understanding of repression. As he struggled to find appropriate concepts he became discouraged over the feasibility of what he was trying to do. He eventually abandoned the project without attempting the intended section on repression. About twenty years later, in his essay The Unconscious, he reviewed the issues he confronted when working on the Project, as follows:

> "If we are to take the topography of mental acts seriously we must direct our interest to a doubt that arises at this point. When a psychical act (let us confine ourselves here to one that is in the nature of an idea) is transposed from the system *Ucs.* into the system *Cs.* (or *Pcs.*), are we to suppose that this transposition involves a fresh record – as it were, a second registration – of the idea in question, which may thus be situated as well in a fresh psychical locality, and along of which the original unconscious registration continues to exist? Or are we rather to believe that the transposition

consists of a change in the state of the idea, a change involving the same
material and occurring in the same locality? This question may appear
abstruse, but it must be raised if we wish to form a more definite
conception of psychical topography, of the dimension of depth in the mind.
It is a difficult one because it goes beyond pure psychology and touches on
the relations of the mental apparatus to anatomy. We know that in the very
roughest sense such relations exist. Research has given irrefutable proof
that mental activity is bound up with the function of the brain as it is in
with no other organ. We are taken a step further— we do not know how
much—by the discovery of the unequal importance of the different parts of
the brain and their special relations to particular parts of the body and to
particular mental activities. But every attempt to go on from there to
discover a localization of mental processes, every endeavor to think of
ideas as stored up in nerve-cells and of excitation travelling along nerve-
fibers has miscarried completely. The same fate would await any theory
which attempted to recognize, let us say, the anatomical position of the
system Cs. – conscious mental activity – as being in the cortex, and to
localize the unconscious processes in the subcortical parts of the brain.
There is a hiatus here which at present cannot be filled, nor is it one of the
tasks of psychology to fill it. Our psychical topography has *for the present*
nothing to do with anatomy; it has reference not to anatomical localities
but to regions in the mental apparatus, wherever they may be situated in
the body."[10] (Freud, 2001, Vol XIV, 173-174)

In the first several lines Freud reviews the difficulty of pairing a
psychological function with a brain region. The abbreviation Pcs stands
for preconscious and refers to things that can become conscious but which
are not yet so, another aspect of his struggle with topography. The middle
lines, especially "But every attempt to go on from there to discover a
localization of mental processes, every endeavor to think of ideas as stored
up in nerve-cells and of excitation travelling along nerve-fibers has
miscarried completely." express his frustration with efforts to correlate
behavioral events with brain events. The last line sums up the position he
arrived at in 1895 when coming to the end of his interest in the Project, for
here he states explicitly that the study of the mental apparatus –
psychoanalysis – has nothing to do with anatomy, at least at that time.

Most of the Project develops around themes of flow of excitation
between neurons and resistance to it. Freud associated flow with lability or
ease of access of one psychic part to another and, since he regarded a flow
as leaving nothing of itself behind, he took unopposed flow to be unable to
result in stored information, this being an aspect of memory and learning.
On the other hand he regarded some neurons as having inherent thresholds

---

[10] Italics in the original.

for flow resulting in a resistance to flow of excitation until the magnitude or intensity of the excitation became large enough, that is, exceeded the threshold. Since such flow could leave something behind and was also associated with a threshold he took this as a sign that such flow resulted in the laying down of information and often referred to such laying down as facilitation, connecting neuronal flow in the context of thresholds with both memory and learning. These ideas are early forms of his yet to come psychological thoughts on the primary and secondary processes.

In his later work Freud regarded the primary process as having two aspects, one relating to emotional lability and the other to cognition. The above idea on unopposed flow foreshadows his later thoughts on the general tendency of the id, or emotional energy and drives, to indiscriminately choose (flow to) objects of potential satisfaction. The cognitive aspect of the primary process, to be developed later, is implicit in this early formulation but only implicit. His ideas on thresholds relate to his later ones on reality testing because such testing requires first learning about the nature of reality in relation to inner needs and wishful tendencies, this being a defining cognitive aspect of the secondary process. The following quotation from the first part of the Project has meaning here:

> "Wishful cathexis carried to the point of hallucination and a complete generation of unpleasure, involving a complete expenditure of defense are described by us as *primary psychical processes*; by contrast, those processes which are only made possible by a good cathexis of the ego, and which represent a moderation of the foregoing are described as *secondary psychical processes*. It will be seen that the necessary precondition of the latter is a correct employment of the *indications of reality*, which is only possible when there is inhibition by the ego."[11] (Freud, 2001, Vol I, 326-327)

The term cathexis was introduced in the English translations of the original German word Besetzung, a noun form of the verb besetzen, meaning to put, lay on, garnish, border, set, lay, occupy or fill. The term cathexis, from the Greek καθέξειν (kathexein) meaning to place, set down or establish, carries the same meaning of residing in or laying in and emphasizes the deposition of a form or excitement or energy – best understood as interest in something in the case of an object or activation in the case of a capacity. Lines one to three of the quotation refer to unopposed flow of excitement, a primary process characteristic. Lines three to five emphasize limiting flow for the purpose of learning as a part

---

[11] Italics in the original.

of the secondary process. The reference to inhibition in the last line is connected with his ideas on certain neurons having thresholds regulating flow.

Some words on historical context will help clarify the meanings here. Freud's model for neuronal communication was based upon his concept of a contact barrier between neurons, this later being named as a synapse in 1897 by Foster and Sherrington. Free flow referred to an absence of resistance or of a threshold between neurons. Freud intuited that an excitation, undoubtedly electrochemical in nature, passed between neurons, carrying information of some kind. The concept of a neurotransmitter electrochemically crossing a synapse did not arise until 1921 with the work of Otto Loewi. Freud's threshold idea corresponds to the build up of an action potential in a neuron that discharges via a neurotransmitter across the synapse.

In general, Freud connected unopposed flow with the primary process and opposed flow with the secondary. The context of his model consisted of complexes of neurons that either stored memories or performed a function as a whole. He regarded the ego as a complex of the latter kind. The phrase network of neurons would do better service than complex of neurons in order to capture the nature of his thinking; as suggested by the current understanding of the phrase neural network. His idea of excitation flowing from one neuron to another implicitly means that the flow takes place along a sequence of neurons of indeterminate length with possibly new branch points (synaptic connections) being formed along the way. It is also implicit that the originating excitation or signal could propagate to more than one terminal point, where a terminal point consists of one or more neurons. In all this, the idea of an association was ever in the background of his thinking, especially in the case of memory. Although his work The Interpretation of Dreams was yet to be written his work with patients up to the time of the Project gave him constant exposure to the role of associating in the formation of dreams, as well as in the formation of symptoms. He felt that the often absurd surface meaning of dreams was a result of a primitive process – hence the term primary process – governing their formation. He said of this:

> "The connections in dreams are partly *nonsensical*, partly *feeble-minded*, or even meaningless or strangely crazy. The latter characteristic is explained by the fact that in dreams the *compulsion to associate* prevails, as no doubt it does in psychical life generally."[12] (Freud, 2001, Vol I, 338)

---

[12] Italics in the original.

He was captivated by his idea of a compulsion to associate as having explanatory power to account both for the formation of dreams and symptoms, but in different ways. In the case of dreams, he felt that the compulsion, when regarded as a propagating excitation carrying certain qualities (emotional meanings) was somehow gathering up images of objects that carry the given qualities to be used in forming the dream scenario. Here the idea of the primary process being weak in differentiation enters because any object carrying the quality will do for purposes of representation, without regard for a real connection to the original significance of the given quality. His model for the formation of symptoms depends more upon another aspect of the primary process, this being unopposed flow or lability. Here a quality (emotion or feeling) inadmissible to consciousness would propagate freely to neurons connected with motor innervation, a concept he felt could account for such hysterical symptoms as paralysis. In the case of non somatic symptoms the above comment on dreams applies, a point to be fully developed later when discussing his finding of the equivalence of dream and symptom formation.. His thinking clearly had one foot in psychology and the other in anatomy. The psychological parts were very much about what appears later in The Interpretation of Dreams, so much so that this work is often regarded as a continuation of the Project.

However, the Project itself was not to be continued. He began with four parts in mind for the final work, the last being on repression which he regarded as the "heart of the riddle" he was addressing. As he struggled with anatomical correlates of behavior in the first three parts he became increasingly disappointed with the feasibility of his ambitious goal. This is reflected in the earlier quote above (Freud, 2001, Vol XIV, 173-174) where he states "But every attempt to go on from there to discover a localization of mental processes, every endeavor to think of ideas as stored up in nerve-cells and of excitation travelling along nerve-fibers has miscarried completely." and " Our psychical topography has *for the present* nothing to do with anatomy; it has reference not to anatomical localities but to regions in the mental apparatus, wherever they may be situated in the body."[13] He reveals this again at a later point in the Project, as follows:

> "Everything that I call a *biological acquisition* of the nervous system is in my opinion represented by a threat of unpleasure of this kind, the effect of which consists in the fact that those neurones which lead to a release of unpleasure are not cathected. This is *primary defense*, an understandable consequence of the original trend of the nervous system. Unpleasure

---

[13] Italics in the original.

remains the only means of education. How *primary defense*, non-cathexis owing to a threat of unpleasure, is to be represented mechanically – this I confess I am unable to say."[14] (Freud, 2001, Vol I, 370)

Despite his disappointments and this discouraging profession, the Project is rich in first formulations of his later and more refined psychoanalytic ideas on the personality, such ideas referring to the primary process and its relation to psychic functioning in general. These later formulations lead to insight into how the personality functions in both health and unhealth, this in turn leading to insight into healing and growth.

The theme of this chapter has been the turning point in Freud's life where he committed his research to a purely psychological approach because he felt that the science and tools of his time could not support the biological or medical approach he was trying to achieve. He accepted that his goal was scientifically premature, but the research perspective it led to resulted in a significant increase and enrichment of his findings. The next chapter begins a presentation of how and why his later understandings of healing and growth, which arose from the subsequent fully psychological approach, are most easily seen in primary process functioning.

---

[14] Italics in the original.

CHAPTER 4

DREAMS, SYMPTOMS AND THE PRIMARY PROCESS

It is surprising that Freud's career path as a researcher, from physician to psychologist, led to a long and significant book on dreams, The Interpretation of Dreams (Freud, 2001, Vols IV and V) rather than to one on psychotherapy, the latter being his main focus prior to writing it. What adds to the perplexity is that only a few years later, in 1905, he published Three Essays on Sexuality (Freud, 2001, Vol VII). Though not a book on psychotherapy it is a book on the psychosexual foundations of health and pathology. With the possible exception of Inhibitions, Symptoms and Anxiety (Freud, 2001, Vol XX) he wrote no books on psychotherapy although he published numerous papers on it. The Interpretation of Dreams (IOD) is usually regarded as his greatest contribution, followed by Three Essay on Sexuality.

He began writing IOD in the late 1890's and finished it in September, 1899, devoting about two years to it. A great deal of thought on the nature of the psyche in both health and illness preceded this work, arising both from his practice and his driven curiosity as to the causes of psychological suffering. His work with patients' associations often led to narratives on their dreams and this was surely a stimulant for his interest. However, it is the events of his life at this time that make sense of why he produced a book on dreams rather than on psychotherapy. It will turn out that understanding dreams is not far at all from understanding symptoms, although he began with only a first understanding of the relation between the two.

Freud's father's death in October, 1896 had a very strong effect on him, so much so that he described the event as uprooting him. In time he came to say that he wrote IOD in response to the loss of his father. Some other forces at play during the writing included his many years of prior research and his deep interest in understanding psychopathology. His uprooting was long lived and the time was coming for his analytic investigations to take himself as their object. Of necessity he began to analyze himself and cites July 7, 1897 as the beginning of his self analysis.

He came to describe it as the most difficult one of all for him. Within it he had to struggle with an upheaval of early and difficult matters of conflict with his father. This means that he wrote his most significant work, the most complete presentation he ever made on the nature of the unconscious, when he was working on his own healing and growth. It is noteworthy here that he came to see his book as a reaction to the loss of his father only as his self analysis came to term.[15] Thus, it will not be surprising to find insights, both explicit and implicit, on the nature of healing and growth in his book on dreams. A reply to why he wrote on dreams rather than on psychotherapy at this time is that IOD builds to an explication of how the unconscious works, a prerequisite both for understanding the neuroses and for psychotherapy itself.

As already noted, the clinical and theoretical material in IOD was drawn both from his work with patients and with himself. This is one reason why many of the dreams interpreted in that work are his own and it also one reason for the large amount of self disclosure within it. He reports that he analyzed over one thousand dreams of patients before undertaking IOD but, fearing bias toward only the case of neurotic dreams, he included many of his own, this having the added advantage of his having potentially full knowledge of all historically determining events that the dream could refer to.

When he began this work he was pregnant with thoughts from the Project, thoughts that predated the loss of his father. Two of the most relevant such thoughts are:

"It is an important fact that ψ *primary processes*, such as have been biologically suppressed in the course of ψ development, are daily presented to us during sleep. A second fact of the same importance is that the pathological mechanisms which are revealed in the psychoneuroses by the most careful analysis have the greatest similarity to dream-processes. The most important conclusions follow from this comparison, which will be enlarged on later."[16] (Freud, 2001, Vol I, 336)

"The aim and sense of dreams (of normal ones, at all events), can be established with certainty. They (dreams) are *wish-fulfilments* – .that is primary processes following upon experiences of satisfaction; and they are only not recognized as such because the release of pleasure (the

---

[15] The phrase 'came to term' is used because Freud's self analysis never ended. He was in the habit of self analyzing at the conclusion of each day. He came to understand the connection with his father's passing when his self analysis clarified him enough to be able to see it.

[16] Italics in the original.

reproduction of traces of pleasurable discharges) in them is slight, because in general they run their course almost without affect (without motor release)."[17] (Freud, 2001, Vol I, 340)

In the second quote he states his early conviction that dreams are wish fulfilments and elsewhere dates his discovery to July 24, 1895. Freud joked about his fantasy of a marble tablet being erected on the spot where he had this insight, the Bellevue Restaurant in Vienna. Jesting aside, this quote adumbrates what he develops fully in his book on dreams.

The first quote refers to conclusions he arrived at after the Project and then presented in IOD. Although most of the book is about dreams, the final section on the theory of the primary process, presents his major finding that the mechanisms for the formation of dreams and of symptoms are the same. In fact he states clearly that the book is building towards this conclusion, as follows:

"The subject to which these dreams of my patients lead up is always, of course, the case history which underlies their neurosis...But these questions are in themselves novelties and highly bewildering and would distract attention from the problem of dreams. On the contrary, it is my intention to make use of my present elucidation of dreams as a preliminary step toward the more difficult problems of the psychology of the neuroses." (Freud, 2001, Vol IV, 104)

The reality behind Freud's discovery that the mechanisms of symptom and dream formation are the same, both leading to the conceptualization of the primary process, is that both lines of investigation were suggesting the same underlying mechanisms. The above quotation, when combined with the one below is evidence of this.

"In venturing on an attempt to penetrate more deeply into the psychology of dream-processes, I have set myself a hard task and one to which my powers of exposition are scarcely equal...Though my own line of approach to the subject of dreams was determined by my previous work on the psychology of the neuroses, I had not intended to make use of the latter as a basis of reference in the present work. Nevertheless I am constantly being driven to do so, instead of proceeding, as I should have wished, in the contrary direction and using dreams as a means of approach to the psychology of the neuroses." (Freud, 2001, Vol V, 588)

---

[17] Italics in the original.

Early in IOD Freud discusses absurdity in dreams and that the laws of
association hold for their formation. This is a prelude to later material on
the principles of dream formation and the role of the particulars of the
primary process. That is, he was preparing the reader for his position that
although dreams appear nonsensical or even absurd, nevertheless, there is
a lawfulness behind their formation.

Also early in IOD he presents examples of dreams that feature images
unknown to the dreamer's consciousness (until verified at a later time). No
doubt he did this because he anticipated his later narrative on the
mechanism of dream formation and the role of early, hidden memories in
their formation. He later returns to dreams that feature images unknown to
the dreamer's consciousness for reasons of morality. He did this to begin
to build to the idea of dreams as fulfilments of blocked wishes, a
connecting link being that the given wishes are seen as prohibited or
dangerous in nature. In this context he reports on the frequency with which
the medical profession has noted similarities between dreams and
psychotic states and notes that Griesinger had pointed out that dreams and
psychotic states have wish fulfilment in common. In the same spirit of
precedent, as well as to motivate later ideas on the inner workings of the
primary process, he notes Aristotle's position that the best dream interpreters
are those who well understand similarity. This paragraph and the prior one
are cited at this point because Freud's presentation of the primary process
occurs late in his book, but is hinted at from the outset.

Some confusion may arise from the fact that although Freud uses the
phrase primary process to refer to the common mechanism of dream and
symptom formation, he also uses the phrase primary processes. The
general use of this last phrase refers to processes that arise early in
development and that lead to other processes, so that here primary refers to
the idea of a precursor to later developments. Similarly, Freud uses the
phrase secondary processes to refer to later processes that serve to regulate
the primary ones in some way. However, the phrases primary process and
secondary process have specific meaning to be developed shortly. Here are
some of his thoughts on these distinctions:

> "When I described one of the psychical processes occurring in the mental
> apparatus as the "primary" one, what I had in mind was not merely
> considerations of relative importance and efficacy; I intended also to
> choose a name which would give us an indication of its chronological
> priority. It is true that, so far as we know, no psychical apparatus exists
> which possesses a primary process only and that such an apparatus is a
> theoretical fiction. But this much is a fact: the primary processes are
> present in the mental apparatus from the first, while it is only during the

course of life that the secondary processes unfold, and come to inhibit and overlay the primary ones; it may even be that their complete domination is not attained until the prime of life. In consequence of the belated appearance of the secondary processes, the core of our being, consisting of unconscious wishful impulses, remains inaccessible to the understanding and inhibition of the preconscious; the part played by the latter is restricted once and for all to directing along the most expedient paths the wishful impulses that arise from the unconscious. These unconscious wishes exercise a compelling force upon all later mental trends, a force which those trends are obliged to fall in with or which they may perhaps endeavor to divert and direct to higher aims. A further result of the belated appearance of the secondary process is that a wide sphere of mnemic material is inaccessible to preconscious cathexis." (Freud, 2001, Vol V, 603-604)

The first sentence refers to the use of the word primary as referring to something being first in time. Freud was thinking in embryological terms where a precursor tissue gives rise to later tissue structures. The second sentence states that in the psychological area there are no known instances of a structure arising without later structures also arising. In the third sentence he states his fundamental thinking that every process must be followed by a later process that serves to regulate it. The remaining lines begin to relate how his thinking on primary and secondary processes connects with his later presentation on symptoms, dreams and the nature of health. As noted the phrase *the primary process* is a specific instance of the idea of a primary process, this being an early one that comes to be connected to a later one. The connection can arise from within so that a secondary process – including *the secondary process* – may evolve out a primary one or it can arise externally to it and come into a relationship with the primary as it (the secondary) unfolds.

For the sake of clarity the presentation will now follow Freud's original sequence of deriving the concept of the primary process, and also of the secondary, from his study of both dreams and symptoms. He often remarked that people, as a rule, fall ill of a frustration. His concept of frustration includes unmanageably strong stress such as over control by parents, because of the child's inability to deal with it consciously and also because such treatment implies that the child was not being well enough loved and cared for, the latter being a frustration in the usual sense. He also had in mind that the onset of symptoms in the adult state tends to be caused by a recent frustrating event so that, for example, a woman who had a frustrating attachment to her father and who recently felt she was failing her spouse could then develop depressive symptoms. All this builds to Freud's repeatedly noting the role of wishful or conative tendencies in the formation of a neurosis.

For both dreams and symptom Freud's definition of a wish was a current in the psyche that aims to replace unpleasure with pleasure. The wish for food when hungry illustrates this as does the wish for companionship when lonely. This definition of a wish in no way suggests how the wish arises nor what the psyche does to fulfil it. When Freud initially worked on this issue he was puzzled by the relationship, if any, between conscious events and dream images that strongly suggests they were somehow connected with those events. A further complicating factor is the issue of how objectionable wishes can be fulfilled. A part of his explanation for dream formation is that waking emotional events that are incomplete continue to be processed unconsciously while awake and that as this proceeds the emotional meanings of the day come to connect with long blocked expression of emotional meanings and strivings from the earliest years. He took this to mean that the waking events activated unconscious emotional trends that have long been blocked, these adding their energy to the initial energy of the waking events. The implicit model here is that the waking experiences lead both to the activation of longstanding, defended against, unconscious ones and to images that can represent the latter within a dream scenario and thus lead to fulfilment. Note how this fits his definition of a wish as a movement from unpleasure to pleasure.

The issue of how these wishes, taken to arise from the id, can be fulfillingly represented when much of their content has long been objectionable to the subject's consciousness is not yet addressed. Indeed, the wishes have been unconscious precisely because of their objectionable nature. Within his model it is mostly the superego that does the objecting, with the ego also taking exception when the wishes are seen to associate with danger or risk, such as a child's initial inclination to express rage with its parents, this presenting the danger of decreasing parental love and putting the child's survival at risk. Freud resolved this problem by defining the ego, the largest part of the psyche, and assigning it the task of creating a dream scenario by working with the id wishes, the superego and reality constraints simultaneously. He referred to the resultant dream images as a compromise formation meaning that the final form of the dream's construction manages to simultaneously give adequate satisfaction both to the id trends and to avoid dream terminating offense to the superego and reality constraints. This arrives at the heart of the problem of the practical task as to just how does the ego in relation to id, superego and reality create the dream. The answer to this strongly involves the use of the primary process. It will help to first present an example to illustrate the model and how it points to the inner workings of the primary process thus far.

A woman who had an emotionally withholding and begrudging mother fails in her attempt to secure a raise from her manager, also a female, although she, the former, felt strongly entitled to it and struggled with her frustration and anger for the rest of the work day. The evening of this event she had a dream in which she saw a beautiful fairy far off, sitting on a high perch and inviting her forward. As she drew closer to her the fairy began to bestow beautiful gifts on her and to praise her. Feeling jubilant she now drew close enough to begin to see the details of the fairy's face and began to tremble. The fairy was transforming into a witch before her eyes, filling her with dread and causing her to run away, leaving the gifts behind.

The dream trigger of her manager frustrating her wish for a raise associates to her mother's emotionally frustrating ways in childhood. Her here and now sense of deserving a raise connects with the childhood expectation of her mother expressing life creating love in response to her needs. The beautiful fairy in the distance is the wished for mother who responds to her needs and the fairy being on a perch connects with the her manager as one over her, just as her mother was once over her. Being invited forward expresses the wish for the motherly attention that she never received enough of. The gifts and praise she receives express the fulfilment of the wish for life creating emotions from her mother. The fact that it is all a wish fulfilling dream enters when the fairy is seen to be a witch, this expressing hate for both the mother and the manager. Her fear and flight express her anxiety over her blocked hate for her mother, and leaving her gifts behind expresses her guilt in reaction to it.

The compromise formation needed for the formation of the dream is between the longing for more motherly support than the woman received in childhood and the expression of the rage that arose from the frustration of that longing. The first form of the fairy and the presentation of gifts and praise enter to satisfy the mother longing but the later form expresses hate for the mother; this turning to fear and dread with abandoning of the gifts expressing how the dream scenario was crafted to stave off superego guilt over the blocked rage trying to assert itself in the dream. That is, the dream satisfies the wish for better mothering but with images that also respect the condemning regard of the superego for the presence of hate; minus the latter the fairy image could theoretically take on a likeness to the mother but in reality this would quickly trigger the intervention of superego guilt to block such imaging because the likeness would bring the dream too close to a conscious experience of the blocked rage and reactive guilt, resulting in the subject waking up to abort the dream. Note that the dream also has a conative trend because of the physiological need for the chronically blocked rage and guilt anxiety to discharge, this need being a part of maintaining biological homeostasis. In a rough sense, the need for homeostasis expresses a physiological wish, connecting it with the dream as a psychological wish fulfilment.

The objects used to create the final dream scenario are an end result of prior work by the primary process on the need to create a wish fulfilling dream subject to superego and reality constraints. The primary process presents now one and then another object as candidates to satisfy both the wish and the constraints. How these objects are selected and how the ego responds to them in the iterative process of dream formation involves the inner workings of the primary process and here Aristotle's position that the best dream interpreters are those who well understand similarity is relevant.

The driving power behind dream formation comes from the activation of a longstanding, frustrated wish (or wishes) from childhood, the wish being a drive or affective tendency arising from the id. Freud conceptualized the id as consisting of instincts striving for discharge via engaging a fitting object. He used the word Trieb, German for sprout, young shoot and motive power rather than the word Instinkt, German for pre-patterned behavior as in the English word instinct, in order to emphasize the impulsive and energetic nature of id instincts. He regarded the primary process as a law of the id characterizing the indiscriminate id choice of objects for discharge. As noted earlier, this has two aspects, one being the lability of instincts, the other being the cognitive choice of object. These two aspects come together upon closer examination of the how primary process works and here Aristotle's words are highly relevant, so much so that it is likely that he had an intuition of the relation between wishes and dreams as well as of the primary process itself.

After the emergence of a wish in relation to an id striving, the next event consists of a series of efforts by the ego to find candidate objects to satisfy the wish. For this series of events to make sense it is necessary to recall that Freud regarded the ego as cortical to the id, meaning that the ego grows from the boundary of the id with interfaces with reality, the superego and the function of satisfying id demands. The subtle point here is that the primary process does specific work in selecting objects, an ego task. However calling the primary process a law of the id makes sense only in light of the ego being cortical to the id because the primary process, by responding to instincts interfaces with the id but by making choices interfaces with ego. This is resolved by locating the primary process on the ego/id boundary. This also resolves the fact that the formation of a wish, although beginning with an id striving, is also a cognitive event and hence the work of the ego.

Freud defined a wish essentially as a transformation that begins with a psychic state of unpleasure and arrives at a psychic state of pleasure. This makes sense in terms of work and emotional energy but it leaves out what a wish *means*, a thing Freud considered to be implicit without often spelling it out. In order to understand how the ego constructs a dream it is necessary to first address the issue of how the content of a wish is used by the ego when invoking the primary process. A wish is defined, for the purpose of dream formation, by its attributes, these being both affective and cognitive. It is important to note that both types of attributes can have highly variable intensities and that this is more often true of affective than cognitive ones. For example the intensity of the affect of affection can be anything from absent to richly present and the same can be said of the cognitive attribute of paying attention. However, the cognitive attribute of being born in a given place cannot have the property of variable intensity whereas that of being blue can.

In the example of a woman who had an emotionally withholding and begrudging mother, the wish could be stated "I wish that my mother would be more endorsing of me and more empathically connected to me." The cognitive attributes are motherly, referred to the self, endorsing and empathic; the affective ones are hope, longing, frustration and anger, the last two implied by the nature of the wish. The work of the primary process requested by the ego – to be formalized later – is to provide objects that have some or all of the given attributes. On a first pass, this ignoring superego and reality constraints, the primary process could offer mother, self and witch, the first two to satisfy the positive affects of the wish and the last the negative ones. The ego, upon receiving such candidate objects would quickly see that the mother as an object is too anxiety provoking to be admitted because it directly links with unmanageable frustration and anger. The witch would be admitted to represent blocked hate because of its ugliness. On a next pass the ego would require the primary process to deliver objects with the given cognitive attributes and with the given affective ones but with lower intensities. This pass could result in the image of a woman with no resemblance to the mother, the self and a witch, the first to stand for the mother and the last for the mother but in a different sense. In the given example the ego could accept the woman as a candidate to represent hoped for mother aspects and the witch to represent the negative, anger related, ones. If the affective intensities associated with the women are strong enough to fulfil the positive and negative longings without violating the constraints then the given objects are accepted as candidates and further work on synthesizing a dream scenario using them is done. If not then further iterations from ego to the primary process take place, this being in the spirit of Freud's frequent comments on the dream work involving a to and fro repetitive process of successive approximations to suitable objects, and then to suitable scenarios using those objects.

For the sake of simplicity and clarity, the example understates how abundantly the primary process actually responds to ego requests for candidate objects. It is to be expected that that the primary process will deliver too many candidate objects because constraints are yet to be considered prior to a second pass and because it is responding to an ego request for objects that carry a few relevant attributes. Thus, the first pass would be likely to result in the set of all adult females to represent the mother, the set of all females of the same age as the woman in question to represent herself and the set of all female villains known to the subject to represent the hurtful aspects of the mother.

In general, a dream begins with the formation of a wish by the joint work of the ego and the id, the latter providing wishful affects and the former responding to their meanings. The ego distils the wish into key attributes and then calls upon the primary process to construct the set of all objects carrying some or all of the given attributes, this done for all attributes of the wish. This begins to hint at the role of similarity in how the primary process works with respect to the selection of objects and at the nature of an iterative process described in the example above where the primary process is called upon repeatedly to deliver objects that meet all constraints.

This will become clearer with further descriptions of how Freud experienced and inferred the meanings of dreams – and symptoms – reported to him. The quote below reveals one of the organizers Freud often used in forming his thoughts on dreams and the primary process:

> "Imagination in dreams is without the power of conceptual speech. It is obliged to paint what it has to say pictorially and, since there are no concepts to exercise an attenuating influence, it makes full and powerful use of the pictorial form....The clarity of speech suffers particularly from the fact that it has a dislike of representing an object by its proper image, and prefers some extraneous image which will express only that particular one of the object's attributes which it is seeking to represent." (Freud, 2001, Vol IV, 84)

The phrase "prefers some extraneous image which will express only that particular one of the object's attributes which it is seeking to represent" refers to how the building blocks of dreams are formed, these being objects which are subsequently used to synthesize a dream scenario. Such objects are selected on the basis of having one or more attributes of the given wish that drives the formation of dream, this clearly tending toward creating images to satisfy the wish, as indicated in the second sentence above. The underlying principle is that of pars pro toto logic, or the part representing the whole, used here in the sense that one or several attributes of an object can be used to represent it and hence by the laws of the primary process, any object carrying said attribute(s) can be used to represent it. That Freud was well aware of this is in the next quotation:

"We have not merely accepted the fact of the looseness of connections in dreams ...but we have shown that it extends far further than had been suspected; we have found, however, that these loose connections are merely obligatory substitutes for others which are valid and significant. It is quite true that we have described dreams as absurd; but examples have taught us how sensible a dream can be even when it appears to be absurd." (Freud, 2001, Vol V, 591)

The idea that one object, say B, can be used to represent another object, say A, because both share one or more attributes is well represented by the words "looseness of connections." For example, suppose that a male with a pronounced drive for success failed to make a connection with a female wearing a red dress. It could then happen that the male would dream the following night of being a Viking with red hair to compensate for the frustration. This illustrates some of the meaning of the phrase "obligatory substitutes for others which are valid and significant" and the phrase "how sensible a dream can be even when it appears to be absurd."

In the spirit of looseness of connections and the role of sharing attributes, Freud commented on a dream he had as follows:

"The phlebitis brought me back once more to my wife, who had suffered from thrombosis during one of her pregnancies; and now three similar situations came to my recollection involving my wife, Irma and the dead Mathilde. The identity of these situations had evidently enabled me to substitute the three figures for one another in the dream." (Freud, 2001, Vol IV, 118)

The idea of substituting three figures for each other based on sharing a similar situation begins to bring to life Aristotle's words on the role of understanding similarity in interpreting dreams as well as to hint at the logical construct within Freud's thinking that these ideas are building to. That construct is further suggested by the quote below:

> "One and only one of these logical relations – *that of similarity, consonance, the possession of common attributes* – is very highly favoured by the mechanism of dream- formation. The dream work makes use of such cases as a foundation for dream condensation, by bringing together everything that shows an agreement of this kind into a new unity. "[18] (Freud, 2001, Vol V, 661-662)

The key line is the first one whose wording indicates that Freud was thinking in terms of *classes of objects*. To be more exact he was thinking in terms of equivalence classes of objects.[19] The word class is used interchangeably with the word set and refers to any well defined collection of objects; however, the word class is usually used to emphasize that its members meet some criterion for membership (as is also true for sets but without the semantic emphasis). The collection of all people with black hair is an example of a set. When a set can be divided using a rule of membership in parts of it, the result is an equivalence relation and in this case it is more common to refer to the set as a class and the subsets (parts) as subclasses. For example, the class of females can be subdivided according to eye color so that all those with blue eyes belong to the same subclass and all those with brown eyes to another. Note that given any one female, she will belong to only one of the equivalence classes (subclasses) so that the equivalence classes do not overlap and are said to be disjoint. Two females with the same eye color are said to be equivalent with respect to the color criterion.

Within the class of all the neuroses, psychoanalysis sees two equivalence classes, the obsessional and the hysteric. The fact that any one actual neurotic will always be mixed obsessional and hysteric does not void this because the label hysteric means that the subject is more hysterical than obsessional and vice versa for an obsessional. Psychoanalysis also sees two equivalence classes within the class of all the psychoses, the depressive psychotic and the schizophrenic. In parallel with the case for neurotics, the label schizophrenic means that the subject is more schizophrenic than depressive psychotic and vice versa. The set of borderlines cannot be further subdivided and has no subclasses, however it remains the case that two borderlines are equivalent as both belonging to the set or class of borderlines.

---

[18] Italics in original.
[19] Italics in original.

The primary process is governed by the concept of equivalence and does great service in describing and accounting for dreams and symptoms, as well as health and creativity, these last two things to be addressed later. Freud felt that the process of dream formation is initiated by emotionally charged events in the waking activity of the day of the dream, including events that can seem trivial. The affective content of such events then begins to connect associatively with defended against, that is unconscious, affective strivings of the same or similar nature. As the day proceeds the activated unconscious trends add more emotional charge to that from the day and this fuels the process of dream formation, from the waking to the sleeping state. The unconscious trends are in the form of wishes, understood to be longstanding but blocked instinctual or affective strivings from childhood seeking release through expression and discharge, things prevented or disallowed by the subject's defenses set in place from an earlier time when such trends were perceived as menacing, dangerous or unmanageable. Within the state of sleep the wishful trends thus activated achieve some satisfaction through the formation of dream scenarios that give veiled or disguised expression to them.

The first major event to occur after the events of the day become connected to unconscious strivings is the formation of the wish or wishes that define them. Any such wish is defined by its attributes, both cognitive and affective but more the latter. Candidate objects for dream formation, delivered by the primary process using some or all such attributes, must carry enough affective intensity to satisfy the given wish but not so much as to cause superego or reality constraints to abort their candidacy. In the iterative process cited earlier the ego calls upon the primary process for objects whose attribute intensities have been modified to maintain satisfaction of both the wish and satisfaction of the constraints. This is clearly a game of deception in that the objects used to create the dream scenario must satisfy the wish without too strongly revealing that this is happening. This becomes clear when the relation of the candidate objects to the changing cognitive and affective intensities, but especially the latter, are examined.

In the example of a woman with an emotionally withholding and begrudging mother, one of the cognitive attributes was motherly and one of the affects was hope. If these were the only attributes used on a first call to the primary process then the resulting equivalence class would be enormous, containing virtually all females known since infancy. It is unlikely that any elements of the resulting class would pass as candidate objects for a dream because superego and reality constraint have not yet been dealt with (in this example) One constraint to be met is that no female be too frustrating because such would run the risk of generating enough anxiety in the dream to wake the subject. A typical ego response at this point would be to call upon the primary process again but with the constraint that the intensity of frustration in any one element be smaller than the first call. This would result in a smaller set of objects, possibly of manageable size for the purpose of dream formation. However, the members of the resulting class must be further examined to see if at least one of the defining wish's attributes is present enough among them to satisfy the wish without violating superego and reality constraints. The iterative process of the ego calling upon the primary process continues until a set of objects that satisfies all constraints is obtained, this being a process of convergence. The resulting set may be excessively large for the practical task of dream formation, a point to be treated later.

The primary process characteristic that emerges from this account is that the size of an equivalence class increases as the number of attributes used to define the wish decreases or as the range of allowed intensities of the attributes widens. This property connects with the feasibility of the ego-primary process interface being able to produce enough objects to meet the defining wish. Similarly, as the number of attributes used to define the wish increases or as the allowed intensities of the attributes decrease the resulting class decreases in size. This property connects with how the task of meeting all constraints decreases the size of the resulting class, part of the issue of necessary convergence already cited.

A dream at one and the same time is a wish fulfilment and also a deception, an oxymoron of sorts made necessary by the fact that while the wish springs from long standing unconscious drives from childhood, its fulfilment is contrary to the forces that made them unconscious in the first place. The fact that a dream is a hallucination suggests its two sided structure as well as nature's reason for evolving the primary process, one side to be seen by the residual of consciousness present in sleep for the sake of wish fulfilment, the other side judging its content with what remains of superego perception and reality testing in the sleeping state to prevent overly strong anxiety or alert that could disrupt sleep. Freud identified three principles that govern dream formation: distortion, displacement and condensation, these doing the lion's share of creating the dream. All three serve to preserve the affective content of the driving wish but to cloak its meaning. All are outcomes of the primary process, a thing made especially clear when the role of equivalence in primary process operation is presented.

Consider here the action of the primary process when summoned by the ego to form an equivalence class of objects carrying specified cognitive and affective attributes of the defining wish that the dream is crafted to fulfil subject to constraints. In general there will be comparatively larger class sizes for any one affect and smaller ones for any one cognitive attribute, because emotional or affective attributes have much lower specificity or differentiation than cognitive ones. For example the affect of hope can be carried by almost anything imaginable, under the right conditions, but the cognitive attribute of being articulate can be carried by comparatively much less because it can only be carried by a person. More extreme in comparison is the class of people whose first initial is H as an attributes of the defining wish. The given cognitive attribute is carried by the defining wish but, since the size of the class of objects that can carry it can be so large, any one member of that class can be very different from objects in the wish, clearly supporting Freud's idea of distortion in object selection and serving the purpose of cloaking the meaning of the dream. At the same time the size of the class of objects that carry a given affect of the wish will also be large making it highly feasible for the ego to choose a member of that class which is quite distant, in the cognitive sense, from objects in the wish, this being an instance of displacement. Note that the selection of members of cognitive classes easily hides their meaning in relation to the wish because any one member may carry other attributes far removed from the qualifying attribute(s) for membership in the class. On the other hand, any member of a class of objects regarded as equivalent for carrying the same affect will carry that affect, regardless of what other attributes it may carry. Hence what the primary process delivers to the ego preserves affect, a necessary condition to satisfy the wish, while also cloaking the affect's meaning.

It can easily happen that a given object belongs to different classes at the same time, this only reflecting that the object satisfies two different equivalence criteria at the same time. For example the class of objects that are green and the class of objects that are shiny clearly have many object in common, such as, for example, a green traffic light. Having one object representing both classes is precisely what Freud called condensation, a thing he felt occurred with very high frequency in dreams. As an affective example of condensation, consider a person who feels hopeful when seeing green objects and who feels anxious when seeing shiny ones. In this example a green traffic light would represent both classes of affect for a driver pressed for time because the driver would hope to make a green light but would also be anxious about not making it, illustrating affective condensation.

The prior two paragraphs demonstrate that the idea of equivalence class formation governing the primary process, when it comes to object selection, accounts for distortion, displacement and condensation. This gives some life to Aristotle's view that the best dream interpreters well understand similarity because any object selected as a candidate for dream formation must carry some attributes of the wish, this making the object similar to the wish. Freud used the term primary process because it is something a neonate is born with and which matures throughout the oral stage, the first stage of life characterized, initially by almost no powers of differentiation at all. Within Freud's model nature made it so in order to expedite discharge of states of excitation, these being mostly affects of pleasure and unpleasure, present at birth (having weak powers of differentiation implies that the given excitation can discharge on almost anything at all). As the primary process matures throughout the oral stage its mechanism becomes increasingly one of equivalence class formation, this being consistent with its initial form where only two classes can exist, those of pleasure and unpleasure, no cognitive classes yet being possible for lack of prerequisite ego powers, with the singular exception of the class of breast like objects. These ideas are summarized in his view that the primary process enables mobility, as presented below.

The central idea is that the primary process manages both choice of objects for discharge and affective lability, the first being a cognitive power and the second an affective power. When the primary process composes an equivalence class with respect to designated attributes it is grouping objects known to the subject that carry the given attributes. However, the purpose of this, in dream formation, is to create candidate objects for inclusion in a dream scenario that results in affective discharge, the fulfilment of the driving wish. The fact that the wished for affects can be made attributes of the candidate objects by the primary process is precisely what lability is, where lability is here understood to refer to easy flow of affect from one object to another; this is also an instance of displacement.

The dream purpose in selecting a member, any member, of an equivalence class is to create cognitive distance from the objects in the dream that carry it. For example, if a single cognitive attribute defining a class is to be round, say, triggered by an interaction with a person having a roundish face, then the class will contain all round objects known to the subject and, if the selected member is a skillet, the cognitive distance from that member to the face that triggered the invocation of the primary process is indeed large. On the other hand selecting class members defined by an affect also works to create distance from the feeling tone or affect in the dream wish because any such member, by definition, will carry the given affect but be different from any object in the driving wish that carries it both by its cognitive attributes, which will tend to differ from those of the wish, and its carrying affects other the defining one for class membership. All this is part of satisfying the dream wish while also satisfying reality and superego constraints on how it is to be satisfied. The use of affective attributes needs to be qualified by the following quotation:

> "Any affect attached to the dream-thoughts undergoes less modification than their ideational content. Such affects are as a rule suppressed; when they are retained, they are detached from the ideas that properly belong to them, affects of a similar character being brought together. " (Freud, 2001, Vol V, 507)

The first line draws attention to the fact that dream distortion tends to leave affects untouched with most of the distortion entering to disguise the meaning of the dream thoughts, things represented mostly, if not entirely, by objects. The remaining lines address a subtle point in which the primary process, in a sense, is invoked upon itself. The idea that affects similar to the initial ones can be used in place of some of the initial ones illustrates this. Here objects carrying attributes similar to the initial ones would also carry some of the initial attributes, a transitive form of similarity. For example, the affect of anger is related to irritability and the latter can replace the former if more disguise is needed to meet the constraints on the dream objects and the scenario they are used to form. As a second example, often found in dreams, the exhibitionistic attribute of being looked at can be replaced by the attribute of looking to hide the meaning of the original one, this resulting in a dream focusing on a viewer rather than on the one viewed.

In the quote below Freud, without directly referring to the primary process addresses the issue of the strangeness of dreams.

> "It has always been a matter for surprise that in dreams the ideational content is not accompanied by the affective consequences that we should regard as inevitable in waking thought...
>
> 'This particular enigma of dream life vanishes more suddenly, perhaps, and more completely than any other, as soon as we pass over from the manifest to the latent content of the dream. We need not bother about the enigma, since it no longer exists. Analysis shows us that the ideational material has undergone displacements and substitutions, whereas the affects have remained unaltered. It is small wonder that the ideational material, which has which has been changed by dream-distortion, should no longer be comparable with the affect, which is retained unmodified; nor

is there anything left to be surprised at after analysis has put the right material back into its former position." (Freud, 2001, Vol V, 460-461)

The first paragraph narrates on the often lack of sensible – to consciousness – connection between the dream images and the feelings they associate with. The second paragraph resolves this with the familiar distinction between the manifest and latent content of the dream, the first being its surface appearance and the second being its disguised meaning. Freud then returns to the lack of sensible connection between the dream as experienced and the affects it gives expression to.

The concept of the primary process arose in Freud's thinking from the recurrence of ideas on similarity in conjunction with ideas on wish fulfilment, in the context of both dreams and symptoms. In fact, within his Collected Works (op cit.) the word wish, and forms of it, occur 1501 times and the word same occurs 3310 times). No doubt many of the uses of the word same occur without reference to wishes but the fact that words related to the word same occur more than twice as frequently as the word wish, a major organizer of Freud's theory, does indicate that thoughts on similarity were also a major organizer in general, and hence include the relation of wishes to dream and symptom formation. This, combined with his explicit emphasis on class membership and the role of attributes to define a class leads to the concept of equivalence class formation as one of the primary process's operational principles or organizers for the selection of objects used in dream formation.

It may appear surprising that the same principle governs symptom formation as well as dream formation for a number of reasons. It is characteristic of symptoms, once formed, to change slowly, if at all over time. Dreams, on the other hand are created on a daily basis and both come and go within minutes or at most hours. In addition, symptoms are experienced almost entirely in the waking state but dreams only in the sleeping state. Yet both are driven by wishes. The wishes behind symptom formation are of the same nature as those behind dreams, both connected with the fulfilment of blocked id drives. The mechanism for the formation of a symptom to satisfy such a wish follows the same principles of distortion, displacement and condensation as dreams; in both dream and symptom formation object selection is governed by the primary process. This leads quickly to the question as to why symptoms do not also change frequently.

Dreams are set in motion by incomplete or unfinished emotional responses of the day of their formation and act somewhat as irritants leading to dream formation once they connect with unconscious and frustrated drives from childhood. Completing the emotional responses is a function dreams have that symptoms do not. In addition the amount of energy available to do the work of dream formation, once asleep, is far less than the amount available in the waking state. Thus, the amount of initial events that can trigger dreams is vastly larger than can trigger the formation of symptoms and, in addition the drive energy that needs to be managed in the dream state is far smaller than in symptom formation. At the same, symptoms arise in order to deal with blocked drive energy in the waking state, making it necessary for the symptom formed to manage much larger intensities of emotional energy than in the case of dreams. The point here is that as dreams are set in motion by daily emotional events that are incomplete, a symptom is set in motion, and held in place, by the presence of strong emotional trends or drive energy in the waking state. This makes it essential for the symptom to have a stability that dreams have no need of and answers the question as to why symptoms do not also change frequently.

Freud's thoughts on the relation between dream and symptom formation are well stated below:

> "It has been worthwhile to enter in some detail into the explanation of dreams, since analytic work has shown that the dynamics of the formation of dreams are the same as those of the formation of symptoms. In both cases we find a struggle between two trends, of which one is unconscious and ordinarily repressed and strives towards satisfaction – that is, wish fulfilment – while the other, belonging probably to the conscious ego, is disapproving and repressive. The outcome of this conflict is a *compromise-formation* (the dream or the symptom) in which both trends have found an incomplete expression.." [20] (Freud, 2001, Vol XVIII, 242)

The words repressed and repressive refer to the use of defenses, probably because the first defense he dealt with at length was repression. The compromise formation refers to the selection of objects and images chosen to simultaneously satisfy both unconscious trends (blocked by defenses) and superego and reality constraints.

The ideas on the primary process and its role in the formation of dreams and symptoms were first presented in IOD and changed little, if at all, throughout the rest of his research. As indicated earlier, it took many years of research, conjecture and modification of concept to arrive at these formulations. His major early biographer, Ernest Jones, who was also an

---

[20] Italics in original

intimate both as friend and collaborator, wrote the following on this point in reference to IOD:

> "The other great trouble was the formidable final chapter on the psychology of dream processes. It is the most difficult and abstract of all Freud's writings. He himself dreaded it beforehand, but when it came to the point he wrote it rapidly "as in a dream." (Jones, 1961, 234)

Jones then adds the following in a footnote, where Ernst is Freud's son:

> "Ernst remembers how his father used to come to meals, from the arbour where he had been writing. "it was as if he were sleepwalking" and altogether gave this impression of being in a dream." (Jones, 1961, 234)

These quotes are cited because the way the unconscious processes emotional meaning is so very different from the way of consciousness – the logic of the unconscious is very different from that of consciousness. The dreamy state that his son cites makes it likely that Freud was struggling with the differences between his conscious versus unconscious understandings of emotional processing. Nonetheless, it will turn out that both modes are distinct instances of a unified model.

All the prior material also connects with what the objects used to form an association are. Such objects are members of equivalence classes and it follows, at least for objects, that an association consists of one or more members of an equivalence class. For example, a person could see images of corn in response to hearing the word yellow; another person might see pencils and daffodils and so on. The full association would, of course, be contained in the verbal narrative that cites the objects.

To digress briefly, the idea that an association consists of members of equivalence classes begins to clarify the use of the term psychobabble. It is used to imply lack of meaning in an analyst's interpretations or associations that arise in response to narrative from the patient. Such associations are members of equivalence classes defined mostly, but not entirely, by the observable, affective attributes of the patient. Finding which of the members makes the most sense psychologically, with respect to the affects involved, is a laborious process and there is no reason to expect first interpretations (analyst's associations) to be accurate. The miss distance involved between interpretation and the patient's psychological reality invites the term psychobabble. However, it also ignores that subsequent efforts at selecting more meaningful members of the equivalence classes usually follow from further interaction with the patient. This is, of course, another example of the idea of convergence.

This chapter has emphasized the role of the primary process in the selection of objects or nouns. The fact that the process depends strongly on equivalences formed on the basis of similarity implies that it can act analogously with verbs. This can be illustrated with the schizophrenic use of language often referred to as word salad. Consider the example in which a schizophrenic is asked "How did you like your meal today?" with the reply "Dishes look good on calendars." The lack of a logical sense in the reply falls away when it is decoded using primary process principles. The object meal belongs to the class of objects defined by the attribute connected with eating; a dish belongs to this class. The object today belongs to the class defined by the attribute of time and a calendar belongs to this class. The verbal phrase look good shares the attribute of being pleasurable with the verb like and hence puts them in the same class. Replacing the nouns and the verb in the reply with the meaning of the classes they belong to decodes the sentence as stating that the subject liked today's meal.

CHAPTER 5

WORKING THROUGH AND THE SECONDARY PROCESS

The primary process has two roles in adaptation, one to promote the discharge of the affective energy associated with id strivings and the second to identify and construct classes with whose members or objects this may happen. Freud usually refers to the first function as one of mobility; the second function is, in a coarse sense, a cognitive one. The mobility aspect means that, given a class defined by attributes associated with an id striving, any, some or all of the elements in that class can be used as objects for discharge of that striving. The idea of mobility is that the associated energy of the striving can be directed to the class elements for discharge via later processing that uses the objects and their energy. It follows that the primary process, left to itself, can discharge along grossly maladaptive lines because of the low level of discrimination with which elements of a class may be selected. This is easily seen in psychotic behavior where, for example, a schizophrenic desiring a cigarette will puff on a piece of chalk because of its likeness in shape and color to a cigarette. This example is based on the fact that the primary process is the dominant mode of mental functioning in psychosis, and this in turn illustrates Freud's summary formula that in psychosis, the unconscious is conscious.

The idea of the unconscious being conscious in psychosis is connected with a form of temporal thinking in Freud. The word primary does indeed refer to the very first developmental happenings in a neonate. At the moment of birth the newborn has a rudimentary primary process capable of identifying the class breast but its great lack of differentiation is seen in the fact that a newborn will try to suckle almost anything soft and roundish. That this initially tiny part of the ego sits on the ego/id boundary is in Freud's idea of the ego as cortical to the id:

> "...we may add that the ego does not completely envelop the id, but only does so to the extent to which the system *Pcpt*, forms it [the ego's] surface, more or less as the germinal disc rests upon the ovum. The ego is not

sharply separated from the id; its lower portion merges into it."[21] (Freud, 2001, Vol XIX, 24)

In the first line he refers to the role of perception (*Pcpt*), anticipating that a greater ego capacity than the primary process will be needed to learn and recognize what things can lead to satisfaction. That the ego does not completely envelop the id refers to the first beginnings of a very basic ego, residing on the boundary of the id. The second line actually states, in alternative words, that the ego and id share a common boundary from which the ego emerges. Freud often referred to this configuration as the ego being cortical to the id, a position that correlates with his view that a major function of the ego, both at the time of birth in first form and more so with later development, is to perceive id impulses and to work to satisfy or fulfil them. He felt that the first issue for id impulses to be satisfied involves the movement of their energy, or mobility, as follows:

> "It will be seen that the chief characteristic of these processes is that the whole stress is laid upon making the cathecting energy mobile and capable of discharge; the content and proper meaning of the psychical elements to which the cathexes are attached are treated as of little consequence. " (Freud, 2001, Vol V, 597)

The word processes refers to all the processes present at birth, a temporal idea, but comes to refer increasingly to his concept of the primary process. The beginning of the first line refers to the need for id energies to discharge, not only for the purpose of adaptation, but also to maintain body homeostasis; Freud implicitly had in mind that if discharge fails to take place then either symptoms will result or a growth inhibiting overload of the personality will. The latter part of the first line directly expresses the indiscriminate and weakly differentiated way in which objects for discharge can be selected. His concern with the need to forestall discharge until object selection has taken place is described as follows:

> "All that I insist upon is the idea that the activity of the *first* ψ-system is directed towards securing the *free discharge* of the quantities of excitation, while the *second* system, by means of the cathexes emanating from it, succeeds in *inhibiting* this discharge and in transforming the cathexis into a quiescent one, no doubt with a simultaneous raising of its level." [22] (Freud, 2001, Vol V, 599)

---

[21] Italics in original.

[22] Italics in original

The phrase *first* ψ-system is a lifting of terms from his Project where the present ideas are given in early form, that is, the *first* ψ-system and the primary process are the same at this point. He states explicitly that there is a need for a second system to keep id discharge at bay, to both await object selection and for the ego to then be better able to direct the mobile energies toward discharge. The second system is, of course, the secondary process. This material is building toward ideas on learning in relation to both the id or emotional satisfaction, and adaptation, these two usually being the same in states of health because the underlying model is that the id's makeup evolved from the long human history of adaptive needs. He begins to describe the development of the relationship of the two processes below:

> "I propose to describe the psychical process of which the first system alone admits as the 'primary process', and the process which results from the inhibition imposed by the second system as the 'secondary process'.
>
> 'There is yet another reason, for which, as I can show, the second system is obliged to correct the primary process. The primary process endeavors to bring about a discharge of excitation in order that, with the help of the amount of excitation thus accumulated, it may establish a perceptual identity [with the experience of satisfaction]." (Freud, 2001, Vol V, 601-602)

The role of the primary process, when it comes to mobility and the regulation of impulsive id trends that it governs, is in the first paragraph. The secondary process not only inhibits discharge but also acts to focus and direct it, this resulting from its cognitive aspect. The phrase perceptual identity is part of what Freud in time called reality sense. The model for the former is that once the ego has found a given object with which to achieve satisfaction via discharge upon it, an image of it is laid down in the ego as a memory. Perceptual identity refers to later ego processing of id demands in which the ego, perceiving available objects for potential discharge, then recognizes that some of them are the same or highly similar to the ones associated with memories of satisfying discharge. At this point the intimate connection between the regulatory and cognitive aspects of the secondary process begins to emerge. Reviewing the developmental sequence from the oral to the anal stage will help make this clear.

The earliest form of the primary process is present at birth. It can form classes of objects that have the attributes being soft, warm and round with a nipple like projection, Once identified such objects are responded to with rooting, this being as aspect of mobility of id energy because it results in the motor action of suckling. Other attributes for equivalence class formation are acquired in the oral stage, one of them being the three month smiling response. Anything resembling a forehead with eyes and nose, including a mask, will elicit a smile from an infant at the average age of three months. There are many other examples of landmark events in the oral stage, each featuring an acquired capacity to discern that an object carries certain attributes; some of this results from a growing capacity to learn and others from innate, preformed sources, such as the recognition involved in the rooting reflex. This is all prodromal to cognitive events that take place during the anal stage as the secondary process unfolds from within the oral, just as does the anal stage from the oral.

Thematically the oral stage is mostly equated with affective events connected with intake. For example, the first thing most infants do when coming upon a new object is to place it in their mouths. People with oral fixations tend to show a greedy eagerness to take things in or to have noticeably large appetites for many of life's offerings, and not just food. This connects the oral stage with an idea of filling up, as in assembling an equivalence class of objects that carry one or more attributes. In addition to this cognitive aspect of the primary process there is also an energic one in the oral stage. Objects selected for class membership must also be able to be made ready for affective discharge, an issue of mobility that precedes discharge. It follows that two major oral themes are intake and generalization, the latter seen in class formation.

As the anal stage emerges from the latter part of the oral, capacities that are complementary to intake and generalization arise. The mobility aspect of class membership, needed to make its members ready for affective discharge, implies that large quantities of affective or emotional energy come to be linked with the class. This is an issue of containment that can be maintained only temporarily because of the risk of psychic imbalance, that is, the need for homeostasis. Like the primary process outcome of the oral stage, the secondary process, outcome of the anal stage has both energic and cognitive aspects. On the energic or affective side, the anal stage sees the burgeoning of powerful forms of aggression, different in character from oral aggression. While the oral form aims at goals of intake, the anal form aims at unfolding toward powers of mastery which, in the healthy state are adaptive and otherwise destructive. Healthy powers of mastery aim to deconstruct what is present into parts in order to reconfigure the resulting raw materials into something adaptive and purposeful; woodworking, from tree to finished product, illustrates this in a clear way. Unhealthy powers seek deconstruction as pleasure in destruction with no sequel of creative or adaptive reconstruction; vandalism is a clear example of this.

The large amounts of affective energy gathered up in forming a class must ultimately be directed into a connection with one or more objects chosen for discharge of the given affective trend and the achievement of its satisfaction. This is an issue of control, that is, mastery. When aggression is understood as the use of emotional energy for mastery, the object of such work can be either within or outside the self, or both. The use of aggression to direct the large amounts of affective energy to an inner representation of an object is an instance of aggression being used adaptively upon a part of the self (preparing for discharge involving the object). This is part of the meaning in the last quote above where Freud refers to the secondary process as both inhibiting and correcting the primary; where his emphasis is on inhibiting discharge while awaiting a suitable time. When the idea of intake is associated with the primary process a form of divergence enters into class formations because many of the objects admitted to a given class will not meet reality demands presented later by the secondary process. In this sense the energic aspect of the secondary process balances the divergent trend of the primary because the secondary process will manage the issue of focusing the large amount of energy distributed over many objects when a class is first formed onto those to be later selected by the corrective aspect of the secondary.

The idea of the secondary process correcting the primary is cognitive in nature. One of the developmental events of the anal stage is the emergence of increasing levels of reality sense. When referred to objects this means the child is becoming increasingly able to see differences between and among objects, an achievement that presupposes both the capacity to learn more attributes and to use them to apprehend which objects carry them versus not. This has dramatic effects on equivalence class formation. In the oral stage, when the number of apprehended attributes is still small, equivalence classes can only be large because many of the attributes needed to distinguish objects have not yet, in general, been acquired. As the number of known attributes increases the sizes of the classes tend to become smaller because of the increased discrimination of objects enabled by the subject's understanding more attributes (the greater the number of attributes, the smaller the number of objects that can carry all of them). This enters a concept of convergence in association with the secondary process in the cognitive sense. Given a fixed object, as the number of its attributes known to the subject increases, the number of equivalence classes it can belong to increases because any such class can be defined using any subset of the object's defining attributes. One the other hand, as maturation proceeds and more attributes of a given object are learned, the size of the class it belongs to, formed on the basis of all its attributes, converges to one. This class of exactly one member, the given object, is the same as the object's inner representation.

When the secondary process is understood in the cognitive sense, it follows that the secondary process is a limiting form of the primary. The generalizing tendency of the primary process, which gives rise to divergence, is supplanted by a convergent process that gives rise to full identification of an object as different from all others. This addresses the closing remark of the prior chapter to the effect that both modes are special instances of a unified model. The basis for unification is that the primary process operates on classes of objects that converge to classes of size one as the capacity to understand enough attributes to distinguish the given object comes forward. A much richer statement can be made: the logics of the primary and secondary processes are the same but the objects on which they operate differ, the former on classes of sizes greater than one, the latter on classes of size one. What's more, the larger the class (and hence the smaller the number of defining attributes), the greater the apparent departure from the logic of consciousness where classes of size one are operated on, the former being pars pro toto logic.

In sum, as the anal stage emerges from the latter part of the oral, capacities that are complementary to intake and generalization arise. The primary process theme of intake, which leads to large amounts of affective energy becoming associated with the members of a class, is moderated by the secondary process theme of focus or direction in which the energy is selectively delegated to specific class members that meet affective constraints unaddressed by the primary process. The primary process theme of generalization, which forms a class of objects that carry given attributes, is moderated by the secondary process theme of convergence, in which objects or members are selected for meeting cognitive constraints as well as superego ones. The affective constraints refer to some affects being too little or too much present in connection with certain members and the cognitive ones refer to some objects carrying cognitive attributes in addition to those specified by the class's definition, an event that can work for or against distortion.

The oral legacy of weak powers of differentiation is the primary process ability to form classes of objects and within its unfolding, to do so with increasingly large numbers of attributes; this oral legacy of generalization begets the power of association because one class member may be used to represent others in the same class. The anal stage legacy of aggression gives rise to the capacity to direct and control affective energy; the emergent cognitive powers of the anal stage result in increasing powers of reality testing.

The oral outcomes form the basis for the mechanisms of dream and symptom formation, as well as fantasy formation and aspects of creativity. The anal outcomes form the basis for the formation of reality sense, as noted, and frustration tolerance. The ability to form classes with only one member is clearly a result of or the expression of the ability to discriminate one object form all others, a cognitive event. However frustration tolerance is an affective achievement that is coupled with a cognitive event. That event is the hard won understanding that delaying satisfaction at one time can lead to greater satisfaction at a later time. Such understanding expands the sense of reality from only seeing objects as potential need satisfiers to seeing the emotional meaning of events that can make them available and then to crafting adaptive strategies to acquire them. This accounting for all the emotional and cognitive content of events associated with securing an object is an aspect of emotional intelligence.

The concept of working through is intimately related to the evolution of the secondary process from the primary. As noted earlier the primary process operates both within the id and at the ego/id boundary. When this is considered in light of the maturational sequence that supports increasing differentiation the concept of the secondary process as a limit of the primary arises naturally. As already noted, the mechanism is that the maturing primary process becomes able to construct equivalence classes based on ever larger numbers of attributes. For any given object it is only a question of time until the process matures enough to form a class based on all the object's attributes, such a class containing exactly one member, the object; this arrives at a secondary process representation of the object. What lies behind this ascent to the secondary process from the primary is something of a quantification of depth into the primary process. This revisits the idea that the smaller the number of attributes to define a class, the larger the resulting class, in general. That is, primary process functioning increases as the number of attributes used to define the class an object belongs to decreases and movement toward secondary process functioning increases as the number of attributes used to define the class an object belongs to increases.

One sign of pathology is a limited ability to discriminate some objects from others, resulting in limited adaptations when such objects are involved. This is a rewording of the fact that some objects that ought to belong, ideally, to a class consisting only of itself, or less ideally, to classes defined by a large number of attributes, in fact belong to classes defined by a small number. This results in confounding of some objects with others, a thing easily seen in transference where the analyst is unconsciously experienced as the patient's father, mother or some other emotionally important person from childhood. In psychosis, where differentiation is very weak, the confounding of objects with one another because of shared membership in classes defined by small numbers of attributes is also an instance where the correlation of the number of the attributes with depth into the primary process is easily seen; it is also easily seen in the odd schizophrenic use of language, often described as word salad. This leads to a rewording of the summary statement at the end of the prior paragraph, that as the number of attributes used to define a class decreases, there is increasingly primitive primary process functioning and, inversely, as the number increases functioning becomes increasingly of a secondary process kind, approaching full secondary process functioning as the number used to define the class increases to the number of attributes any one object carries. This dependency on the number of attributes makes both primary and secondary process functioning relative to the objects involved and implies the familiar situation where a person may be high functioning in some areas while being low functioning in others at the same time.

The motivation to work through arrives when the subject appears to have a first cognitive and somewhat emotional understanding of a significant unconscious issue. Working through has two aspects, one aiming at emotional change and the other at structural change. The first is the often long and labored work of creating the ego strength in the subject to begin to deal consciously with long blocked unconscious affective trends, usually involving childhood frustrations and often involving rage reactions, abandonment anxiety and so on. The accuracy of the analyst's interpretation, the degree to which the analyst experiences what the subject cannot yet experience emotionally because of defenses and low ego strength as well as the analyst's supportive presence, are all major factors in bringing about the desired emotional change. Within this context healing is understood to be the removal or undoing of psychic states or processes that generate symptoms and limit adaptation. Growth is understood to be the emergence of adaptive powers as blocked material is liberated, this resulting in the previously blocked drives becoming free to resume the growth that was always intended by nature. These emotional or affective events of healing and growth are easily observed in the subject because of symptom reduction and the joy of newly emerging capacities.

Such observation, while satisfying for the both analyst and subject, does not tell on the inner structural changes taking place in the latter.

Evidence of healing and growth in the structural sense is found in some specific changes in the way the cognitive aspects of the primary and secondary processes are altered. A major connecting link between the affective and the cognitive is in the way the processes represent and select objects both for dream and symptom formation, and in the ordinary work of adapting. To begin with an example, suppose that a young woman was raised by a mother who was overly indulgent and who had black hair and a highly attentive way. The young woman when taking a course as part of her professional responsibility experiences anxiety while in it. The unconscious dynamic issue is that the young woman felt, as a child, that her mother was failing to endorse her as an autonomous person, leading to rage reactions and hence to guilt. The class teacher is a woman with black hair and who, in the role of a conscientious teacher, had to be attentive, all three factors promoting an unconscious perception of the teacher as the mother and leading to a re-experience of the anger and guilt issues with the mother. In equivalence class terms the class defined by woman, attentive, black hair contained both the mother and the teacher (as well as many other objects) and the inclusion of both led to the anxiety symptoms.

Looked at more closely, the example illustrates a primary process property that could well be described as inheritance, a consequence of the primary process operating on the basis of similarity. The fact that the teacher and the mother shared some attributes inclined the woman to unconsciously experience the teacher as her mother and this resulted in anger and guilt, and hence anxiety reactions to the teacher. Put differently, the teacher inherited some of the affective attributes of the mother. The term inheritance is used to describe an unconscious dynamic that is usually referred to as distortion and/or displacement; however inheritance emphasizes that members of a class can be treated by the primary process as if they had attributes carried by other members of the same class, in addition to those used to define membership in the class. Dealing with this therapeutically involves both healing and growth issues. One healing issue involves the work to undo the teacher inheriting the negative affective attributes of the mother because they do not, in reality or in health, belong to the teacher. This event leads to the removal of the teacher from those equivalence classes of the mother that are defined using the attributes of anger and guilt (as well as possibly others). One growth issue, in the case of the woman, involves adding more of the attributes that truly belong to the teacher to her representation, such as being conscientious. Note that this means adding attributes to the teacher as a member of any class

containing her, regardless of how the class membership attributes themselves
are selected. Note also that this addition will, in general imply that the
teacher comes to belong to new classes whose defining attributes include
those in the addition. As noted in Chapter 4, any one object can belong to
more than one class, and in general, will [23] and therefore the healing work,
or working through, would result in some, possibly all, of the classes
containing the mother, the woman or the teacher being modified as
indicated.

An affective gain would take place if the analysis succeeds in
diminishing the woman's anger with her mother, an event seen in a
decrease of the intensity of the affective attribute of anger in the woman's
representation of her mother. Note here that this does not add an attribute
to the mother but diminishes the intensity of one already defining her. As
therapy proceeds and the woman's anger subsides it is entirely likely that
she will then become able to see more of the real attributes of the mother,
especially the positive ones, this leading to the addition of attributes to the
mother's representation.

The term working through is fitting for the primary and secondary
processes because all unhealthy attributions of all relevant objects must be
undone and healthier or more actual properties of such objects must be
added to the way their class memberships are defined. It is also fitting for
the desired affective changes because such things are achieved piecemeal
and rarely, if ever, all at once. What both cognitive and affective change
have in common is being connected with objects. The emphasis here is on
the fact that the affective changes result in clearly identifiable changes in
the attribute dynamics of the primary and secondary processes, these being
ultimately numerical in nature, some being removed, some being added,
some featuring changes in intensity. The ability to experience stronger or
weaker levels of already present emotions or feelings is a connecting link
between cognitive and affective change because affective processes can
both inhibit and facilitate cognitive ones.. However the major significance
of affective change is in the capacity to experience either previously
blocked feelings and emotions or completely new ones, the former being a
variety of healing and the latter a variety of growth; this is, in fact, the
vernacular meaning of therapy.

---

[23] For example, a red apple belongs to each of the five classes defined by the
following single attributes: red, fruit, roundish, tasty and nutritious. Each of these
five classes clearly contains objects different from a red apple. For example the
class of things that are red includes a red airplane. A red apple also belongs to the
class defined by the two attributes: red and nutritious which contains the very
dissimilar items beef, tomato sauce and strawberry icing.

The removal of an inherited attribute from an object in a class does not remove the object from the class because it still retains the original attributes that define class membership. However, the removal brings its representation, closer to reality, this being a step in the direction of a secondary process representation where it will eventually belong to a class consisting of only itself; before this happens the object is represented in a way that confounds it with others because it can then only belong to classes with more than one member. On the other hand, adding appropriate attributes to an object is a clear secondary process gain in the sense of approaching, and possibly achieving, enough attributes to distinguish the given object from all others. The cognitive aspects of working through can thus be summarized as removing inherited attributes from objects, a weak gain in secondary process representation, and the addition of realistic attributes, a strong gain. A full working through corresponds to these events taking place for all the classes that each given object belongs to. A full working through implies that the subject has increased realistic representations of objects and is thus able to make more realistic emotional and cognitive decisions for solving presenting life problems.

Removing inherited attributes can appear, at first glance, to limit creative adaptation because it could be argued that some attributes, though inherited, may yet be appropriate for the inheriting objects, but this is not so. By definition when an attribute is inherited it is added to an object without the review or evaluation of the secondary process. It follows that the ego cannot yet use the inherited attribute in an adaptive sense. As for creative adaptation, the inherent power of the primary process to choose objects with weak connection to some known objects is preserved by the nature of healing and growth. That is, the mechanism of using attributes of some initial objects to gather up more objects also carrying those attributes is unaltered. In the case of dream and symptom formation this means that the resulting classes have received minimal secondary process review but in the case of waking adaptation or unconscious creative work, the classes are scrutinized for the degree to which they represent reality or can give rise to feasible recommended solutions. This can be summarized by stating that inheritance takes place before secondary process review.

The concept of working through is intimately connected with the concept of transference because the majority of any one analysis is working through and the majority of working through takes place during transference. The word comes from the Latin preposition trans, meaning across and the Latin verb ferre meaning to carry or bear. The present participle of ferre is ferens, leading to the construction transferens which translates as carrying across. The etymology goes quickly to the central meaning of transference, that a patient in analysis soon comes to experience the analyst as emotionally significant figures from childhood such as father, mother, siblings and so on; this perception is mostly, but not only, unconscious, especially in the early phase of analysis. The analyst's perception and interpretation of the patient's transference and dreams leads to a deepening understanding of the early emotional forces that shaped the patient. This also leads to an increasingly clear understanding of the patient's defenses, all this leading to the ongoing work of interpretation to undo defenses and build ego strength as the once defended against material gains access to consciousness. This raises the two questions as to what is ego strength and what is the nature of emotional health.

Ego strength, in a loose sense, is the power to adapt, often with emphasis on frustration tolerance. More exactly it is the ability to bring forward all of one's available capacities in response to the need to adapt to a presenting challenge. It is the opposite of such terms as falling apart or caving in. Its full meaning is seen in the opposite sense in the phenomenon of schizophrenic fragmentation where even mild demands result not in a coordinated adaptive response but in a regressive dedifferentiation of the personality. Ego strength, in an ideal sense, refers to the ability to allow the personality to form an orchestrated response to a challenge that can invoke all relevant healthy capacities already in place. It implicitly contains the ability to hold the course where further growth is needed for a sufficient adaptation, this relating it to frustration tolerance.

Freud felt that the major signs of a person being healthy are in the ability to love and to work. Evidence of these two criteria occurs in identifiable changes in the primary and secondary processes as the subject's health increases. The fact that work and love are not independent within the personality but interrelated makes the evidence easier than otherwise to see because their interdependence amplifies the signs of healing and growth and hence results in more signs of primary and secondary process change.

It is not just by design that psychoanalysis drives a subject to revisit childhood but it is also in its very nature to do so. The subject comes to analysis seeking relief of symptoms that, unknowingly to the subject, bear upon both the fulfilment of early wishes and their frustrations. The given parts of the personality leap out to the analyst as the arrival of the wished for parent who will provide love where it was in short supply and life creating emotions that were in short supply in childhood. In other words, transference is inevitable because the unrequited longings of childhood respond to the analyst as a promise to fulfil those lifelong yearnings.

The most basic of all childhood longings is the wish to be fully certain of being loved and wanted. This, together with a supportive and permissive environment will result in a psychologically healthy child; failure to do both will result in a damaged personality. If the failing figure is the mother then the burgeoning equivalence class of females will forever after carry the attributes of being frustrating, a source of pain and being untrustworthy, among many other possibilities. Within the transference the subject will unconsciously experience the analyst as both the frustrating and the wished for mother. Working through at this point is a matter of interpreting the subject's perceptions and experiences of the analyst, as well as others, in order to begin to remove mother attributes, mostly negative, from the subject's equivalence class definition of females. Although this reduces the number of attributes that describe the given class and may appear to be an increase in primary process functioning, it is actually a movement toward secondary process functioning because of the removal of erroneous or unrealistic attributions to females. At the same time the working through process adds attributes to females, including the mother, that went previously unseen because of defenses thwarting their perception and processing. This increases the number of attributes for the given females and is also a movement toward more secondary process functioning. In sum and in the context of love, working through removes erroneous attributes and adds correct ones to certain classes. These changes, in the case of a successful analysis, enable the subject to more objectively perceive the mother and other females as lovable or unlovable figures. The same kind of remarks apply to issues arising from early relations with the father.

Working through as a matter of interpreting the subject's perceptions and experiences of the analyst and others, in order to begin to remove inappropriate mother attributes, concerns attributes that have variable intensities, as is always the case with affective ones and sometimes the case with cognitive ones. If the quantification or intensity of a given unrealistic attribute includes all levels, then objects carrying the given attribute will be dropped from all the classes in question. If the level is specified as greater or less than a certain amount, then the object may or not be dropped depending on the intensity it carries; finally if the level is specified as between a minimum and maximum level, then the object may or not be dropped depending on the intensity it carries. In all cases the levels referred to are those achieved after a therapeutic effect has taken place, so that class membership for the given attributes is decided upon the basis of the new levels, more aligned with reality, and no longer the original ones. In the last three of the four cases, some primary process functioning may or may not be preserved, though if preserved, it will be reduced, moving the subject, with respect to the given objects, closer to secondary process functioning.

It is to be emphasized that the noted process changes are cognitive, or object defining, in nature because all such changes involve logical decisions based upon intensity. They are the result and sign of healing and growth in the affective aspects of the processes driven by the work of interpretation and the nature of the analyst's expressed emotion. Interpretations tend to build conscious connections between what is unconscious and what can be seen or experienced in awareness, this leading to more evolved processing of long standing blocked trends from childhood. The analyst's role is more than just that of an interpreter. An interpretation given formula-wise and without the analyst having sufficient emotional experience of its meaning will have little effect on the subject. On the other hand, when the analyst sees and also emotionally experiences the meaning of the subject's state, the subject's emotional system is, in a sense, invited to participate in that of the analyst, an event that tends to promote affective healing and growth. This involves the capacity for resonant empathy between subject and analyst as well as the analyst's support and scientific understanding of how the personality functions in health and unhealth. This therapeutic aspect refers to the affective changes in the processes, an increase in relevant mobility within the primary and an increase in focusing power for the secondary, matters to be discussed in the next chapter.

The other part of Freud's summary that equates health with the ability to love and work is implicit in the quote below:

> "The child's parents, and especially his father, were perceived as the obstacle to the realization of his Oedipus wishes; so his infantile ego fortified itself for the carrying out of the repression by erecting the same obstacle within itself. It borrowed strength to do this, so to speak, from the father, and this loan was an extraordinarily momentous act." (Freud, 2001, Vol XIX, 34)

The idea of the child fortifying its ego by borrowing strength from its father has much to do with how a child learns the ways of life from its parents. The central meaning here is that a child senses how its parents respond emotionally to various presentations from life, both big and small. When a child has a similar presentation it will either recall how its parents dealt with it emotionally or, if it is the case, how they deal with in the present moment. In both cases the child feels the same or similar emotional stirrings as its parents and these, by the very nature of what emotion is, began to prepare the child for taking action to deal with whatever is presenting. This means that the child learns how to work by watching how his parents work and then repeating in himself what he senses they felt when dealing with a task. It also means that the parental affects felt while dealing with the objects of a task become attributes of the objects themselves, facilitating later adaptations based on miming what the parents did both emotionally and in motor action.

Before such things take place a child will feel curiosity and helplessness as well as frustration and anxiety in response to a task it cannot manage. Such affects are repeated in the transference situation, quite strongly with oedipal transference, to be discussed later. Pre-oedipally, the subject will present with such affects over life challenges that were experienced as either incomplete, or worse, as unmanageable. The working through issue at this point is the undoing of the attribution of helplessness and anticipated frustration and anxiety to objects that carry such themes. For example, suppose that a man had a competitive and aggressive father who made him feel as a child that he was inept and could not measure up. He reports in his analysis his strong anxiety over the need to master a software system at work. The analyst senses the anxious feeling of helplessness in the subject and its relationship to his reaching out for a fatherly demonstration of how to deal with the work situation, the latter being a carryover from childhood frustrations in being shown how to manage life tasks, both the skills and the affective instilling of confidence. A number of issues arise. The analyst knows that satisfying the subject's wish to be shown how to deal with his dilemma will not work because it is only in childhood that satisfying an infantile wish can lead to growth; satisfying such demands after childhood leads not to growth but to repetition of the demand, often with escalation, as well as to infantile clinging and dependency, opposites of the therapeutic goal of autonomy. Rather the wish needs to be frustrated to break down the subject's defenses so that blocked rage over the early deprivations can begin to approach awareness and so that consciousness may be slowly prepared to deal with it. The desired affective changes in the way the subject deals with the work issue will lead to a number of identifiable changes in the primary and secondary processes.

Within the transference the subject will unconsciously expect the analyst to be competitive and aggressive as his father was and to treat him as if he cannot resolve his work issue. Interpretive work regarding the resulting feelings of helplessness and frustration, when effective, will result in the subject's attributions of the analyst shedding some of the father ones, or if the attributes are quantified, in their intensities falling, a movement toward more secondary process functioning. The subject's own attributes will see a decrease in the intensity of the affects of helplessness and a rise in those of competence, the former mostly a decrease in primary process functioning and the latter an increase in secondary process functioning. Assuming effective therapeutic work, the subject will experience some of his previously blocked rage and the associated guilt reactions to it, implying a decrease in the subject's attachment to the wish for more life promoting fathering than he received in childhood. This will manifest as a decrease in the affect of father longing, a movement toward more secondary process adapting, and a movement away from the attribution of omnipotence to the father, this being an increase in reality testing and a secondary process gain. The intensity of the affect of rage as a father attribute will diminish as will the intensity of guilt in self attribution, and these signs of healing and growth will be reflected in less primary and more secondary process adaptation. The fall off in guilt will lead to more positive attributes in connection with the various representations of the self as well as with objects of interest to the subject (because unconscious guilt would work against the perception of positives).

Much of the inherent connection between transference and working through arises from the analyst being an attractor for all unresolved early relationships. Each in their turn, serially or simultaneously or both, are created anew or repeated as their attributes are called forth by the transference to then become attributes of the analyst within the patient/analyst interaction, this inviting interpretation and working through. The approach can properly be called a bottom up approach for a number of reasons. The fundamental goal of analysis is to bring about emotional change, a thing that implies change in how instincts and their derivatives become attributes of objects in both the primary and the secondary processes. The former, instincts and their derivatives, emerge earlier than most primary process object choices and much earlier than most secondary process ones. Since development proceeds from precursor forms to descendant forms it is fitting to call this a bottom up sequence.

It has been implicit that therapeutic change as reflected in the primary process tends to take place earlier than in the secondary, mostly because the first exists before the second begins to emerge. This too fits a bottom up model. More exactly as healing takes place one expects the loose generalizing tendency of the primary process, to treat similar objects as the same thing, to abate as objects become more emotionally distinguishable or differentiated. As growth takes place one expects the inner representations of relevant objects to acquire more attributes, these being appropriate, so that the only object carrying all such attributes is the object itself, a class of one. This describes how healing and growth move from inappropriate primary process representations both to more realistic primary representations and to the limiting form of secondary process ones. The companion changes in mobility for the primary process and in focus for the secondary are treated in the next chapter.

This part of the bottom up concept helps to clarify some of what Freud had in mind when he said that psychoanalysis is about making the unconscious become conscious. An evoked response from the personality begins with unconscious perceptions followed quickly by primary process classification of their component parts or objects based on their first perceived attributes. The response then propagates upward toward a secondary process response and hence into consciousness where some, usually not all, secondary process events are perceived. This describes events in a healthy response but in a neurotic one there is a failure of some of the primary responses to propagate into secondary ones. Making the unconscious become conscious in the neurotic case means, in part, removing the obstacles to propagation. That is, making the unconscious conscious sees the previously indicated changes in primary and secondary process functioning take place; such changes being observable in attribute assignments to objects. The bottom up concept also accommodates the fact that one of the strongest criteria of health is spontaneity because the first evoked responses in adaption are unconscious, whether or not they can propagate into consciousness, as in the healthy case where the conscious perception is also spontaneous or freely received rather than thwarted by defenses. This is not to say that primary process mobility propagates into secondary process functioning but rather that sufficient affective flow, or spontaneity, is also a health criterion outside the primary process.

To a small degree there is also a top down approach in analysis, although it is the preferred method in most non-dynamic forms of therapy. A top down approach begins with a recognition of a maladaptive strategy in the subject, followed by the analyst suggesting a more adaptive one in the hope that the subject will be able to shed the former and begin to live the latter. There is little, if any effort, to identify or deal with resistances within the subject to moving from the maladaptive to the more adaptive relation to life, in the given area. The analyst here hopes that suggestion and support will be able to result in the affective changes needed for the transition to take place. Where the bottom up approach seeks to get affective and cognitive attributes into more realistic connections with objects, the top down approach suggests behavior whose realization requires such connections to be made. This is likely to work when the subject is labile enough or when defenses have been sufficiently weakened. The idea of urging the subject on to better adaptations by spelling them out is not new to analysis and, in fact, Freud occasionally did so.

Within either approach it is ultimately defenses that hold up the necessary healing and growth that enable affects or drives to become connected to appropriate objects, this being a matter of realistic or healthy attribute assignment. The very role of defenses is to keep affective material that was early on perceived as dangerous or unmanageable away from awareness and away from those parts of the psyche that can communicate enough with consciousness; such material and parts include primary and secondary process representations of objects. Undoing of defenses is a premiere goal of any dynamic or bottom up approach. However, within successful dynamic psychotherapy a time arrives when the given healing and growth is soon to take place and it is at such a time that the top down approach is likely to succeed because support and directive counsel can well provide the incremental energy needed for the healing and growth to now take place. The present view is that the top down approach can probably accelerate the final phases of the bottom up approach in any one targeted therapeutic area.

Evidence of any one defense weakening occurs in the suggested changes in primary and secondary process functioning and representation. A giveaway sign of a reaction formation is insufficient lability. Although the symptoms in an obsessional are governed by the primary process, much of the adaptive use of the primary process in generalizing is weak in many emotional areas or even not present at all in some. Such generalizing is a prerequisite for eventual convergence to a secondary process representation of an object because of the need to add more attributes to the definition of any one class, some of these arising as inherited attributes belonging to the added members. It is also needed to support general lability in the personality. The evidence for outgrowing this weakness is close to the surface because when the given changes occur the subject will express more affective attributes in either responding to or in defining various objects. The movement from over-generalizing via emotional attributions that equate objects based on shared feelings to secondary process precision is similarly close to the surface. Some telltale signs of this would be a decrease in the use of affective attributes and an increase in the use of cognitive ones. The other part of a reaction formation, within an obsessional, is the overcompensated expression of the opposite of the blocked rage, seen in excessive compassion, politeness, helping and so on. A sign of healing and growth in this part of a reaction formation would be a decreases in the size of equivalence classes defined by single attributes such as compassion, politeness and helping.

Repression is a defining defense in hysteria that seeks to keep feared affects from being connected with objects that have access to awareness. This is also true of a reaction formation, when it comes to rage, but the extent of the repression's effect on objects is small compared to that of a reaction formation, the latter setting in earlier than the former. Behavioral evidence of healing taking place – the lifting of the repression – is the onset of flooding as a result of sufficient weakening of the defense of repression, an event that also takes place with the weakening of all defenses.[24] A typical use of repression would be to keep the affect of seductiveness, in a male, away from the attributes of his mother and sisters. First process evidence of the repression weakening would be a rise in the intensity of consciously felt `seductiveness in response to other females, followed by the onset of mild intensity of it in relation to his mother and sisters. In the first case, other females, the size of the primary process class defined by seductive female would increase and in the second, the attribute of seductiveness would be added to those of the single member classes defined by mother and each sister. These events are similar to those in the case of the undoing of a reaction formation because healing and growth must always see decreases in primary process functioning and increases in secondary. However, the degree of developmental arrest associated with a repression in hysteria is far less than that with a reaction formation in the case of an obsessional. These observations on the processes accord well with Freud's view that obsessional expressions are a dialect of hysterical ones, the dialect being the lesser use of affect and the greater use of cognition in the obsessional.

The defenses cited above are dominant in the neuroses. Merging is a common defense in the psychoses as well as in the borderline personality. It is often cited as a clear example of primary process functioning. Loosely speaking, merging is motivated by an inner need to feel filled up with more life, as in depressive psychotic states where deficient internalization of the mother as the good object leads to painful feelings of emptiness, often distressing enough to lead to wish fulfilling hallucinations of life givers and to end of the world delusions. Merging enters as a defense against such a painful state by inclining the subject to lose the sense of

---

[24] When an obsessional improves there is a shift away from obsessional behavior toward hysterical behavior, the downgrading of the neurosis moving toward an hysteria. It is often comical to observe how an obsessional, upon improving and entering hysterical flooding with the weakening of his reaction formation, reports that he is getting worse!

difference between self and another, this enabling the subject to regard many parts of the other, especially the other's vital processes, as also belonging to the self. The result is the addition of objects carrying the attributes of these parts and vital processes to the primary process classes of the self. This is not the same event as inheritance unless some members of the class of the self already carry those parts as attributes. The addition of such parts to the class definitions of the self to create the feelings of the life of the other being also in the self is a primary process event often associated with dedifferentiation of the self as well of the self and the other. Dedifferentiation, or loss of psychic structure and of the ability to distinguish between different objects, means that the number of attributes used to define the self, as well as other objects, diminishes in order to make the class of the self equivalent to more objects, especially the object defined by the person being merged with. This is a deep, or highly primitive, level of primary process functioning.

The therapeutic goal here is the restoration of the differentiation between self and other, a non trivial therapeutic task for both the analyst and the subject. Signs of success in this endeavor are not initially the shedding of class members admitted in the defense of merging, but rather the addition of more qualifying attributes to the primary process classes containing the self, this being a movement toward secondary process functioning and its power to distinguish objects from one another.

In general as the work of psychotherapy lifts defenses there is a movement away from primary process functioning toward secondary process functioning. This applies at both the affective level where maladaptive mobility decreases and adaptive mobility increases as well as to the cognitive level where differentiation of objects increases. It also includes the point where both affective and cognitive gains meet, this being the joint increase in reality testing and frustration tolerance. This segues into the next chapter where another kind of relation between the processes arises, the present one being the oral legacy of mobility and generalization with the anal one of focus and object discrimination. Where working through achieves more efficiency within the first two processes and an adaptive relationship between them, working through in the next stage sees a refinement and increase in a third process that characterizes the way humans adapt.

CHAPTER 6

HEALTH AND CREATIVITY:
THE TERTIARY PROCESS

There are five psychosexual stages within Freud's model, these being oral, anal, genital, latency and puberty. The first three are regarded as building to a final foundational form that can support all later growth; the analogy with the frame of a building to which all later parts are added is fitting. Since the third stage ends approximately by the fifth year of life Freud felt that it is not possible to damage the personality after about that age. His point of concern was that a child can be hurt, that is made to suffer psychologically, after that age but damage to the central or foundational form cannot occur after that age as a result of behavioral factors.

Although he felt that an infant is born into the oral stage with the primary process already in place, he nevertheless saw the primary process as an outcome of the oral stage because of its growth and maturation within that stage: it is one of the components of the foundational form. As noted previously is that he saw the secondary process as an outcome of the anal stage and he regarded the highly differentiated affective and cognitive powers of the secondary process as complementary to those of the primary. He also saw the primary process as having a mobility function, meeting the need to bring emotional energy to various tentatively selected objects in preparation for action and saw the secondary process as having a focusing function for the given energy, also preparatory to action but with much greater resolution of what the objects of the given adaptive response should be.

Freud did see the third or genital stage as having outcomes but he did not identify a structural component of the personality in the same sense as the primary and secondary processes being oral and anal outcomes respectively. More to the point here, he did not do so explicitly. The issue of the third stage having outcomes but not an explicitly identified foundational component within his model becomes clearer when the stages as psychosexual events are examined. A first issue is the meaning of sex or sexual within his model:

"In psychoanalysis the concept of what is sexual comprises far more; it goes lower and also higher than its popular sense. This extension is justified genetically; we reckon as belonging to 'sexual life' all the activities of the tender feelings which have primitive sexual impulses as their source, even when these impulses have become inhibited in regard to their original sexual aim or have exchanged this aim for another which is no longer sexual For this reason we prefer to speak of *psychosexuality*, thus laying stress on the point that the mental factor in sexual life should not be overlooked or underestimated. We use the word 'sexuality' in the same comprehensive sense as that in which the German language uses the word *lieben* [to love]. "[25] (Freud, 2001, Vol XI, 222-223)

The first line draws attention to the wider than nominal understanding of sex in psychoanalysis. Its extension to tender feelings remains within the nominal understanding but its extension to *anything* derived initially from sexual drives is a point of departure. A fuller extension is the inclusion under sexuality of drives which originated as sexual in nature but transformed their aims or goals into nonsexual ones; sublimation is one example of this and the excitement a person can feel upon studying a work of art another. It is implicit in his use of the word psychosexuality that he is concerned with the relationship of sexual drives to the formation of ego powers to satisfy them, a point of great relevance to what he saw the first three stages as building toward. Comparing the use of the word sexuality to the use in German of lieben draws attention to Freud regarding all forms of pleasure as sexual in nature. This last point still gives rise to confusion as it did in his own era because of the tendency to equate sex with genital activity. Though not stated above Freud's idea of sex also included the idea of survival, both individually and collectively, the latter easily seen in reproduction. These points are elaborated in the following:

"This much may be said by way of a general characterization of the sexual instincts. They are numerous, emanate from a great variety of organic sources, act in the first instance independently of one another and only achieve a more or less complete synthesis at a late stage. The aim which each of them strives for is the attainment of 'organ-pleasure'; only when synthesis is achieved do they enter the service of the reproductive function and thereupon become recognizable as sexual instincts.... They are distinguished by possessing the capacity to act vicariously for one another to a wide extent and by being able to change their objects readily. In consequence of the latter properties they are capable of functions which are

---

[25] Italics in the original.

far removed from their original purposive actions—capable, that is, of 'sublimation." (Freud, 2001, Vol XIV, 125-126)

Freud's model for the sexual instincts sees them as a diverse group that emerges at first from organic sources and initially without a relatedness to each other. Lacking such (eventual) relatedness they do not yet seek pleasure in a general, shared choice of an object but find pleasure in relation to themselves; for example within scoptophilia pleasure is taken in looking without connection to, say, contrectation, an instinct for touching. The sexual nature of these instincts is not easily seen at first but becomes clear later when they come together to serve reproduction. Their lability and tendency to easily change one object of satisfaction for another implicitly refers to the primary process, some of this supporting sublimation.

His thoughts on the structure of the sexual instincts and their eventual goal are presented in next two quotes.

"We find ourselves on firmer ground when we investigate the manner in which the life of the instincts serves the sexual function. ...It is not the case, then, that we recognize a sexual instinct which is from the first the vehicle of an urge towards the aim of the sexual function – the union of the two sex-cells. What we see is a great number of component instincts arising from different areas and regions of the body, which strive for satisfaction fairly independently of one another and find that satisfaction in something that we may call 'organ-pleasure'. The genitals are the latest of these 'erotogenic zones' and the name of 'sexual' pleasure cannot be withheld from their organ-pleasure. These impulses which strive for pleasure are not all taken up into the final organization of the sexual function. A number of them are set aside as unserviceable, by repression or some other means; a few of them are diverted from their aim ...and used to strengthen other impulses; yet others persist in minor roles, and serve for the performance of introductory acts, for the production of fore-pleasure." (Freud, 2001, Vol XXII, 97-98)

Freud emphasizes that the sexual instincts do not emerge fully formed for the task of reproduction but rather emerge as a set of component instincts that first emerge without much, if any, relatedness to one another, as noted earlier. It is an interesting but relevant aside that when he states "What we see is a great number of component instincts ... which strive for satisfaction fairly independently of one another" he is unknowingly building on prior ground. In medieval theology human nature was regarded as in a corrupted state such that each of its faculties sought its own immediate end without regard for the others. This state, referred to as concupiscence, was seen as a fall from a higher state in which all the faculties worked collaboratively toward joint fulfilment or satisfaction. The relevance here is that the medieval view emphasized conflict, a key part of the Freud's view of the causes of pathology. The analogue of the higher state within Freud's model is that the genitals, being the last to mature sexually, support the goal of reproduction. This is not to make theology of psychology but rather to emphasize that the inner knowing of these sexual structures is so basic as to result in formulations that carry that same structure but in a different context, a point considered to be of a veridical nature because we can only express what we are. As for the components themselves that fail a later integration with fully genital aims, some are defended against with resulting adaptive loss while those not defended against are acted out or lived as perversions, some are sublimated and others can serve the preparatory role of fore-pleasure.

> "Manifestations of the sexual instincts can be observed from the very first, but to begin with they are not yet directed towards any external object. The separate instinctual components of sexuality work independently of one another to obtain pleasure and find satisfaction in the subject's own body. This stage is known as that of auto-eroticism and is succeeded by one in which an object is chosen." (Freud, 2001, Vol XIII, 88)

While much of this quote repeats what has already been said, the added point is that sexual satisfaction begins narcissistically directed at one's own body. The idea of an object eventually being chosen for genital satisfaction in the service of reproduction anticipates events in the third, genital stage.

Freud saw the sequence of psychosexual stages as building toward an increasingly adaptive personality. Within his model there are implicit ideas on accumulation of adaptive capacity from one stage to the next and there are explicit ideas on the evolving capacity for a person to love, the latter being strongly about movement out of narcissism and toward loving significant others, if not mankind as a whole, this said despite Freud's low regard for much of humanity. [26] At issue here is that while Freud saw both structural and adaptive gains in the first two stages, he saw more of structural gains than of adaptive ones in the third stage. This is presented in the context of his position that a person is healthy if that person can work and love. His implicit references to third stage adaptive gains and problem solving need to be considered to clarify the relations of the first two stages to the third one. Some narrative on what he saw as the structural gain in the third, or genital, stage will begin the discussion.

---

[26] This, no doubt, being one reason for his fondness of Mark Twain.

He regarded genital primacy as a major outcome of the genital stage. The component instincts that emerged in the first two stages now move toward an integration or synthesis that strongly supports the goal of reproduction. One consequence of this integration, in the ideal case, is that the component instincts no longer act independently of one another but act in unison. Another consequence is that sexual excitement culminates in genital discharge regardless of where it originated on one's body. In the real, or non–ideal case, some component instincts are either only partially integrated or remain outside the integration, this forming a basis for perversions; partially integrated components can support mild perversions. A salient difference between the role of component instincts in the perversions and in genital primacy is that the former take pleasure often without aims connected with love or reproduction and with objects that are both human, including non-genital body parts and non-human, whereas the latter takes pleasure in reproductive aims and often with love, and in a state of health, always with love. In the quote below Freud narrates on the roles of integration and of an object in both cases.

"...I wrote that 'the choice of an object choice, such as we have shown to be characteristic of the pubertal phase of development, has already frequently or habitually been effected during the years of childhood: that is to say, the whole of the sexual currents has become directed towards a single person in relation to whom they seek to achieve their aims This then is the closest approximation possible in childhood to the final form taken by sexual life after puberty. The only difference lies in the fact that in childhood the combination of the component instincts and their subordination under the primacy of the genitals have been effected only very incompletely or not at all. Thus the establishment of that primacy in the service of reproduction is the last phase through which the organization of sexuality passes.

"Today I should no longer be satisfied with the statement that in the early period of childhood the primacy of the genitals has been effected only very incompletely or not at all. The approximation of the child's sexual life to that of an adult goes much further and is not limited solely to the coming into being of the choice of an object. Even if a proper combination of the component instincts under the primacy of the genitals is not effected, nevertheless, at the height of the course of development of infantile sexuality, interest in the genitals and in their activity acquires a dominating significance which falls little short of that achieved in maturity." (Freud, 2001, Vol XIX, 141-142)

The idea of the third stage building to the choice of an object, that is, a person to love, and of genital primacy being approximately complete in childhood are precursor ideas to what Freud regarded as a fundamental event in the third stage. In pregenital life the component instincts are drawn to objects on the basis of need satisfaction; there is no question of the instincts looking to edify or satisfy the objects they choose. The coming together of the component instincts into genital primacy enables a child, for the first time in its life, to also love on the basis of what the object is rather than only on the basis of what needs it can satisfy. This large turn away from narcissism toward object love for what the object is finds full expression in the Oedipus complex. Freud felt that the complex begins around age three and is characterized by a child developing a possessive longing for its opposite sex parent with anxiety over how its same sex parent will respond to such overtures. This leads to jealous rivalry with the same sex parent and, in the case of the male, leads to castration anxiety. Events are similar in the case of female but here castration anxiety is replaced by evisceration anxiety in which the little girl unconsciously dreads that her mother will punish her by removing the anatomical ability to replace the mother as child bearer. Both genders fear punishment by losing the love of their same sex parent. Both genders feature an ambitious wish to replace their same sex parent. The child's idea of what this means is limited to the understanding that the parents have a special meaning to each other and that it is somehow expressed by sleeping together. The child's position or hope is that whatever that special thing is between the parents, the child wants to take on the role of the same sex parent in it. Ambition, rivalry and possessiveness are the hallmarks of the Oedipus complex.

` It is a given that no child can ever actually succeed in winning its oedipal wish; it is simply impossible. This leads to the question as to what nature is up to in making an impossible urge come upon the child in the first place. Freud offered a partial answer to this in his formulation that the superego is the heir to the Oedipus complex. His starting point is that somehow a child comes to eventually accept the utter impossibility of what it wishes for. Freud saw the final outcome of the oedipal attachment in the ethical area. What follows refers to the usual heterosexual oedipal attachment; the issue of homosexual oedipal attachment will be discussed later.

However charming a little boy's possessive love for his mother may be, he must still reckon with the inherent conflict of having to regard his beloved father both as a rival and a possible menace. To make matters worse, the boy will tend to unconsciously study those parts of the father that please the mother in order to clone those parts with an eye toward making better offerings to his mother; this complicates the healthy identification with the father already underway from the anal stage. While in the oedipal drama the child is diligently crafting strategies for winning by using the ego capacities acquired in the pre-oedipal stages. Such strategies must be evaluated not only for prospects of success but also with respect the dual risks of losing his father's love and drawing his father's anger upon himself. Such considerations are new to the child and also engage the ego powers emerging in the genital stage, these being related to ambition, success or winning, risk assessment and, ultimately, feasibility. While it is true that Freud saw the Oedipus complex as very much about ambition his dominant view was how it influenced superego formation and hence his view that the superego is the heir to the Oedipus complex. The child learns to restrain or somewhat abandon his oedipal wishes to avoid punishment, a lesson in the superego inhibiting behaviors and strivings judged harshly by its father, possibly also by its mother. That is, the ethical issue is that the resulting superego becomes able to internally control aspects of oedipal behavior by generating guilt and fear. As in his general model for superego formation, the child internalizes its parents' values and becomes regulated from within as it was at first regulated from without. Freud emphasized the role of castration anxiety as a theme in the formation of the superego in the third stage, this being clearly connected with fear as a moderating factor. His following eventually saw that the analogue of castration anxiety in the female is evisceration anxiety, as already noted. What both genders have in common is fear of loss of love of the same sex parent as a result of oedipal strivings.

There is little in Freud's writings, at least of an explicit nature, on what capacities the ego grows in the genital stage in the pursuit of success and conflict resolution. His noting that the wish for oedipal triumph or victory is doomed to failure from the outset connects superego formation to the management of frustration but says little, if anything, about what powers the ego grows to deal with the inherent conflict and still less about how to try to make success happen. However, he noted that the ego tends to turn strongly to sublimation of the objectionable drives and regarded this as one of the pillars of civilization. It is worth noting here that sublimation involves the use of the primary process because the blocked drives find expression in things associated with their original aims. For example, a boy's blocked longing for his mother's affection could be sublimated into entering a caring profession because the equivalence class defined by the attribute of being affectionate includes caring professions; similarly a girl's blocked longing for her father's assuring presence could be sublimated into entering a profession requiring leadership, such as executive work because the equivalence class defined by the attribute of being assuring includes executive presence. Nevertheless, Freud's major explicit insights surround how the child's experience of the entire oedipal drama influences its pursuit of success in life in general. In other words, Freud studied the impact of the Oedipus complex on motivation. His position on this is made explicit in the following quotation:

> "Even a person who has been fortunate enough to avoid an incestuous fixation of his libido does not entirely escape its influence. It often happens that a young man falls in love seriously for the first time with a mature woman, or a girl with an elderly man in a position of authority; this is clearly an echo of the phase we have just been discussing, since these figures are able to re-animate pictures of their mother or father. There can be no doubt that every object-choice whatever is based, though less closely, on these prototypes." (Freud, 2001, Vol VII, 228)

The header in the original that immediately precedes the above is "After Effects of Infantile Object-Choice", at which point Freud has been narrating on how the third or genital stage builds to the choice of a love object, the mother in the case of the male and with the female, the father. He addresses the idea that the object choices made in the oedipal attachment become a model or prototype, for better or for worse, in the subject's later choices. This means not only that a new object choice will have certain resemblances, both affective and biological to the original but also that the dynamics of the interaction with the new object will be much like the original ones. This led him to investigate the role of the oedipal attachment in the subject's later efforts at success, both attaining it and fearing it. At another point, and in a similar vein, he writes:

> "The sexual behaviour of a human being often *lays down the pattern* for all his other modes of reacting to life. If a man is energetic in winning the object of his love, we are confident that he will pursue his other aims with an equally unswerving energy; but if, for all sorts of reasons, he restrains from satisfying his strong sexual instincts, his behaviour will be conciliatory and resigned rather than vigorous in other spheres of life as well." (Freud, 2001, Vol IX, 198)

Although he begins here with sexual behavior he soon connects success in the area of sexual love with the likelihood of success in other areas of life and, inversely, connects failure in that area with failure elsewhere. His narrative is hinting at some form of prototype or canonical form in relation to creating success. That his findings on success address more the issue of motivation than of possible mechanisms operative within a prototype is in the following:

"I have, however, already remarked elsewhere that if a man has been his mother's undisputed darling he retains throughout life the triumphant felling, the confidence in success, which not seldom brings actual success along with it." (Freud, 2001, Vol XVII, 156)

This quote does not directly link the general ability to create success with the Oedipus complex but it is not far from it either. It notes the connection between creating success and pleasing one's mother, though in the case of a female pleasing the father could be a stronger issue. Freud developed the general idea of post oedipal pursuits of success being perceived, at the level of motivation, as repetitions of oedipal competition and fear of punishment at many points. Thus, while the quote relates to positive aspects of motivation to create success, Freud's works on success are mostly about the unconscious equating of pursuit of success with oedipal ambition and therefore to what tends to inhibit the creation of success.

The possessive ambition that characterizes the Oedipus complex is the first significant other oriented pursuit of success in every person's life, and for both genders. That it should lead to a prototype at both the motivational and structural levels would not then be surprising. Before shifting the narrative to the evidence for a structural or mechanistic model for the creation of success within Freud's thinking, another kind of oedipal attachment needs to be addressed.

Within the oedipal triangle a male child has a first of its kind loving attachment to his mother which triggers fear of loss of his father's love as well as castration anxiety. These are emotions and fears of an intensity it has not previously experienced. It can, and does happen, that the stresses become too much for the boy to manage, this leading to another way to live out the strong oedipal attachment. The other way is to take the rival father as the oedipal object, enabling the other-centered emotional dynamics of the complex to be lived. The boy unconsciously senses that doing so staves off the fear of losing his father's love and punishment, the latter sometimes being more a presumption rather than a perception.[27] The boy's love for its mother regresses, to one degree or another, to his pre-oedipal attachment to her. The homosexual attachment to the father involves the parallel to the usual oedipal attachment, the issue of how to win the oedipal object. One strong aspect of pre-oedipal love is identification with the mother. Within the

---

[27] Freud speculated that oedipal dread of punishment is phylogenetic because of the extent of its occurrence and the presumption that the complex has been repeated in an evolutionary time frame, that is, a very long time.

regression away from her as the oedipal object is the prospect of learning something of the art of seduction from her, for she had first claim on his father. The outcome is a homosexual object choice whose strategy is based on cloning some of the ways of the mother, a root of the characteristic femininity in most homosexuals. Freud referred to this an inverted Oedipus complex and regarded homosexuality as neurotic. That this was something of a problem for him, in light of his position that everyone is born bisexual, is something he never addressed. It is now known that homosexuality, in either gender, can be biologically driven and not just neurotically. Having noted this, the issue here is that whether the oedipal object is the mother or the father, an ambitious pursuit of the love object takes place and this involves the problem solving matter of how to win.

The oedipal triangle for a female is similar but with some significant differences. The little girl feels an inward turning toward the father in a new way, the attachment to the father beginning pre-oedipally and need based around age two. In parallel with the little boy she wishes to love her father possessively more for what he is than for the needs he satisfies and wishes to have him respond in kind. Other-centered love begins to emerge within the oedipal attachment and the girl begins to see her mother as a rival with fear of losing her love and of being punished by her for her wish to take her place. Ambition and the wish to triumph over the mother arise. If anxiety associated with the mother's response is overly strong and/or if the father is made overly anxious by this attachment the little girl may resolve the anxiety issue by withdrawing her oedipal interest in her father and directing it at her mother. Symmetrically with the boy she wishes to seduce the mother as she once wished to seduce her father. The retreat from the father regresses back to an identification with him in which she can study and learn some of the ways that make her mother want him, with an eye toward doing the same for herself. While the oedipal attachment to the father was still operative the girl would similarly be studying the mother for what about her makes her father prefer her, the copying or miming of this forming part of the oedipal strategy that she later renounces in the inverted case.

Freud emphasizes that the usual oedipal attachment for the girl is a more difficult psychological task than for the boy because there is a change in gender from the pre-oedipal mother attachment to the oedipal love for the father. He felt that this is one reason for females having more emotional intelligence than males. He also felt the sameness of gender in the homosexual attachment of the girl to her mother, together with the mother being the girl's first attachment, account for the more accepting attitude of society toward female homosexuality in comparison to males. As with the little boy, whether or not the oedipal attachment is inverted, it involves an ambitious pursuit of a love object and presents the first other oriented problem solving task of large significance in the child's life.

Freud saw the genital stage as giving rise to the Oedipus complex and to the final form of a foundation for all later growth of the personality. This contrasts with the structural outcomes of the oral and anal stages, these including the primary and secondary processes. It is implicit in his narrative that the child uses both the capacities of the first two stages as well as newly emerging ones in managing its oedipal attachment. However, his discussion of third stage capacities only visits the motivational aspects of the attachment and not the emergence of new capacities. Yet his position is that the third stage results in something of a final form for all later growth. In addition he notes that post oedipal efforts at creating success tend to follow the oedipal model, so that the degree of success in the latter is predictive of the general level of success in all later endeavors. What's more he was strongly interested in culture and creativity but far more from the perspective of motivation than the inner structure or form of the creative mechanism. The emphasis on object pursuit and the wish to triumph, or create success within the oedipal attachment suggest that there are structural third stage events not explicitly identified in his model. But there is evidence in his writing that he implicitly identified outcomes of such events and that the sum of such outcomes builds to a third stage outcome that has been called by some, but not by Freud, the tertiary process.[28]

To understand what can form an implicit third stage outcome it is necessary to review some other aspects of Freud's thinking on the nature of the unconscious. The word itself has a number of different meanings and uses, ranging from its role as an adjective to the naming of a part of the psyche or one of its capacities. For example, the statement that dreams take place in an unconscious state is an adjectival use of the word. On the other hand the part of the psyche that does the work of creating a dream forms a part of the ego whose functioning cannot become conscious, except in psychotic states. In all cases when the word unconscious is used as a name it is to identify a psychical region whose functioning cannot, in states of health, occur in awareness but whose products may be able to enter awareness. An ordinary example of this occurs when a person suddenly sees a solution to a problem. Here the solution is the end product

---

[28] Highly notable is the work of Arieti, Creativity: The Magic Synthesis (Arieti, 1976), where he presents material on the nature of creativity from many different perspectives, including the mechanistic one.

of processes that take place unconsciously and which cannot fully take place consciously, except perhaps in psychotic states.

The issue being addressed here is that much psychical work, both for adaptation and against it in pathology, takes place in unconscious systems and that a number of such systems participate in such work. Freud's work on identifying some of the unconscious systems that perform the work of pathology is familiar, but the use of such systems in the work of adaptation much less so. The quote below is given as a transitional link from the unconscious work that precedes dream formation to unconscious work that takes place before an adaptation:

> "It remains for us to give a dynamic explanation of why the sleeping ego takes on the task of the dream-work at all. The explanation is fortunately easy to find. With the help of the unconscious, every dream that is in process of formation makes a demand upon the ego – for the satisfaction of an instinct, if the dream originates from the id; for the solution of a conflict, the removal of a doubt or the forming of an intention, if the dream originates from a residue of preconscious activity in waking life. The sleeping ego, however, is focused on the wish to maintain sleep; it feels this demand as a disturbance and seeks to get rid of the disturbance. The ego succeeds in doing this by what appears to be an act of compliance: it meets the demand with what is in the circumstances a harmless *fulfilment of a wish* and so gets rid of it. This replacement of the demand by the fulfilment of a wish remains the essential function of the dream-work."[29] (Freud, 2001, Vol XXIII, 169-170)

In the first three lines Freud draws attention to the ego as a problem solver when he uses the phrase "every dream that is in process of formation makes a demand upon the ego." In the fourth line the ego again enters as a problem solver with respect to the wish to remain asleep. Lines five and six then describe some of the work that the ego does in solving the given problems. In point of fact Freud saw the ego as evolving out of the id in order to manage the id's needs or demands; that he also saw the ego as interfacing with both reality and the superego in doing so further lays it down as a problem solver. That the ego is using both the primary and secondary processes, and a something more, will be addressed later. The problem solving theme for the ego appears more strongly in the next quote:

> "We have so far been studying dream-wishes: we have traced them from their origin in the region of the *UCS*, and have analysed their relations to

---

[29] Italics in the original.

the day's residues, which in their turn may either be wishes or psychical impulses of some other kind or simply recent impressions....It is not impossible, even, that our account may have provided an explanation of the extreme cases in which a dream, pursuing the activities of daytime, arrives at a happy solution of some unsolved problem of waking life."[30] (Freud, 2001, Vol V, 564)

The first sentence describes some of the mechanisms the ego uses in dream formation. The second sentence directly expresses the possibility of the dream work arriving at solutions of ordinary problems arising in waking activity. The next quote takes this idea further:

"If a dream carries on the activities of the day and completes them and even brings valuable fresh ideas to light, all we need to do is to strip it of the dream disguise, which is the product of dream-work and mark the assistance rendered by obscure forces from the depths of the mind...; the intellectual achievement is due to the same mental forces which produce every similar result during the daytime." (Freud, 2001, Vol V, 613)

The obscure forces that "even bring valuable fresh ideas to light" include the primary and secondary processes. The last two line states explicitly that the mental capacities that result in an intellectual achievement within a dream are the same as those that do so in waking life. The idea of unconscious capacities producing solutions to waking problems is again stated explicitly below:

"I know that it is asking a great deal, not only of the patient but also of the doctor, to expect them to give up their conscious purposive aims during the treatment, and to abandon themselves to a guidance which, in spite of everything still seems to us accidental. But I can answer for it that one is rewarded every time one resolves to have faith in one's own theoretical principles, and prevails upon oneself not to dispute the guidance of the unconscious in establishing connecting links." (Freud, 2001, Vol XII, 94)

The first sentence is in the Zen spirit of the need to give up attachment to what does not work well enough or not at all in order to become able to see what can work better. It is direct counsel on the need to release attachment to conscious processing, when it is insufficient, in order to more fully open to unconscious processing. That such processing can achieve more than known conscious contents is directly stated in "...prevails upon oneself not to dispute the guidance of the unconscious in establishing

---

[30] Italics in the original.

connecting links." The links referred to are those that begin with the understanding of a presenting problem and terminate with elements of a solution to it that are generated by unconscious processes.

The present position is that dream formation is a solution to a problem, this being a need for long standing, blocked instinctual trends to find expression and hence a reference to Freud's description of dreams as wish fulfilments. However, dreaming takes place in children before the beginning of the third or genital stage. If, as is to be suggested, the third stage gives rise to a tertiary process that supports general problem solving in adaptation, then what does one make of its predecessor, the dream making mechanism? As outlined earlier, a dream is created by a part of the ego that visits and revisits both the primary and secondary processes for objects that can enter as images for wish fulfilment subject to the constraints of the id, from which the wish arises, of the superego which enters moral constraints and of reality. This ego function must involve the powers of both perception and evaluation in order to perform the indicated work. Prior to the genital stage these powers function only, or mostly, to create a wish fulfilling scenario, an event that is entirely intra-psychic. Freud's narratives on the third stage are devoted almost completely to the arrival of the Oedipus complex as a defining event for that stage. The event does involve inner drives but the problem to be solved involves an object relationship, this being the ambitiously possessive love for the child's opposite sex parent, in the nominal case. A first level of difference between the invocation of the given ego powers, in their pre-oedipal forms, and those in the oedipal form is that the former can only involve narcissistic object relationships, whereas the latter sees a strong other oriented object relationship that has non-narcissistic parts. A parallel between the two is that in dream formation the ego must resolve superego constraints and, while this is also true in the oedipal attachment, it must also resolve reality constraints such as what will the opposite sex parent make of the child's overtures as well as issues of general social and cultural pressure that the child senses. Put differently, the oedipal attachment sees the beginning of the ego working to solve strongly emotionally charged problems that involve outside the self objects, both personal and otherwise.

The given ego powers are used for the task of dream formation, both before and after the Oedipus complex, and in this sense its pre-oedipal form can be called task specific. When this is considered in light of Freud's positions that the personality achieves an essentially final foundational form by the end of the third stage and that as the Oedipus complex goes, so do later efforts at success, the idea of the third stage resulting in a general problem solving power or mechanism suggests itself as being implicitly present in his thinking all along. This arrives at the sometimes considered idea in psychoanalytic thinking of the third stage resulting in a tertiary process of some kind related to the need for a general problem solving mechanism.

It is not accurate enough to say that as the anal stage emerges from the oral stage or that the genital stage emerges from the anal. The onset of the genital stage can occur while the anal stage is still emerging from and being integrated the oral. In addition, the inherent tendency of the psyche to unify as it evolves and grows suggests that the genital stage arises when the integration of the first two stages are well enough, though not yet completely, formed. Well enough formed means that some ego capacity has emerged to enable sufficient coupling of the primary and secondary processes to support dream formation. This something is not a third stage event but a precursor to it found in part of the mechanism of dream formation described earlier. To recapitulate, a dream begins with the stirring of a wish derived from long standing and frustrated wishes from one's earliest years, usually cued by waking events in the day of the dream. Note that the fact that children dream is consistent with this even though one usually regards dreams as occurring later in life.

The first task of the dream maker is to identify the affective and cognitive attributes of the wish with an eye toward invoking the primary process to form classes of objects that can satisfy various subsets of the attributes. The secondary process is then invoked on these first pass results to identify which objects in the classes either do not adequately satisfy the affective longings in the wish or satisfy them too much and hence violate some superego constraints. It is further invoked to examine the objects to determine if any affects not in the wish but contrary to the superego constraints are attributes of any of the objects. The first pass results in a winnowing down of candidate objects for a dream scenario. A second pass follows and is treated similarly and as many passes as needed are made until a set of objects that well enough carries the attributes of the wish and well enough meets superego and reality constraints is formed, these being a set of objects to be used to create a dream scenario. The dream maker works under the strong constraint of satisfying a wish but not so much as to stir superego driven anxiety that can result in violating the other first task of the dream maker, to keep the subject asleep; note that the dream is perceived by the residual of awareness in the sleeping state. Though not essential for the current discussion, it is worth noting that one adaptive result of the dream is the expression, and hence discharge, of blocked emotional trends in the personality, a thing necessary to maintain homeostasis of the personality and the biological processes that support it. Such discharge is, in part, an effort to bring the blocked parts of the personality nearer to consciousness for assimilation and, in this sense, it can be argued that one function of dreaming to slowly weaken defenses against such healing and growth taking place.

Within the work of dream formation prior to the creation of a dream scenario several distinct forms of work are carried out. The first task is identifying the attributes of the wish that drives the dream in the first place. This may sound like it presupposes full linguistic ability but the fact that young children dream points to an earlier ability that is a precursor to the emergence of language, the latter taking place at the average age of eighteen months. Before a child can use symbols to represent feelings or ideas, it uses objects. A preverbal child could, for example, use the image of a red rose where at a later time it would use the symbol 'red.' This is easily seen in dream formation itself where it is altogether typical for a regression from words to objects used to represent them takes place. A part of the pregenital ego senses the stirring of a wish and then, using what of the secondary process then exists, gathers up its identifying attributes. The next task invokes the primary process, as indicated above, and the complimentary invocations of the secondary, also as indicated above. Iterations follow and the final step, for present purposes, is the creation of a set of candidate objects for a dream. This is not a repetition of the prior paragraph as it may seem because the same kind of work becomes a subset of later work done when the tertiary process emerges in the genital stage. The work described thus far is done by what can be properly called the dream maker, an ego function or capacity that is a precursor to the tertiary process.

The tertiary process arises in the context of the Oedipus complex, an event that Freud took as defining much of the genital stage. The expansion of the dream-making precursor to this process has a number of distinguishing features. The precursor is invoked to solve only one kind of challenge, to satisfy a wish. This is an entirely intra-psychic event. At first the tertiary process, arising in conjunction with the challenge of winning the oedipal competition is crafted in part to solve a single problem, but it is a problem of unprecedented complexity for the child and involves both intra- and extra-psychic objects and events. That it is surrounded by charming childish fantasies reflects that the early phase of the tertiary process is little differentiated from the dream maker with a strong dependency upon the primary process and a still weak dependency upon the secondary. Unlike the wishes that drive dreams and have a life cycle of a day or less, even though the same wish may recur at later times, the oedipal wish is sustained for a long time, approximately from age three to somewhere between ages four and five. There is a pressure to perform, that is, to make something in the way of success happen, that is not present in dream formation, the former resulting in expressed behaviors and inwardly felt experiences, the latter resulting only in images and felt experiences. The emerging tertiary process has a far larger responsibility than its precursor, to which it adds the roles of active, conscious relatedness to objects outside the self.

Freud was fond of identifying psychological processes that function as prototypes for later, similar processes. For him the Oedipus complex was the prototype of the pursuit of success, but only with regard to motivation in his explicit discussions of it; the issue of mechanism was implicit. That he did not also explicitly present tertiary process mechanisms (or even name such a process) is surprising given the rich detail with which he identifies the mechanism of dream formation. The largest step in the mechanistic direction occurred when he saw that the mechanisms for the formation of dreams and symptoms are the same even though symptoms always involve active, conscious relations to both self and non self objects, a thing dreams can only do in the most indirect way through the relations of the driving inner wish to external objects connected with the creation of the wish. This sets the stage for the function of the third process to be general problem solving.

There are many pregenital problem solving actions in a child, as seen in its emerging motor skills and its emotional cueing of its parents or caretakers. Examples are found in its play with toys, its efforts to reach what it wants or to signal that it wants to be held or fed. A pregenital child can even cue its parents or caretakers into seeing that they are frustrating it. None of the early problem solving involves either the emotional complexity or the strong risks of the oedipal challenge. Early problem solving usually involves the relationship of motor skills to the secondary process, including the emergence of some logical abilities, and the relationship of the primary process to the quest for alternate objects of satisfaction, an option not present in the oedipal attachment (unless a regression occurs). These early gains are precursors to the tertiary process because they involve managing an emerging relationship between the primary and secondary processes and also because such management is subject to achieving a goal with respect to an object relationship, where the object can be a person, a plaything or an aspect of the self. In the case of healthy development the emotional demand placed upon the child slowly increases as it moves through the pregenital stages, and the precursor becomes able to respond to increasingly intense emotional challenges, these being increasing levels of both excitement and frustration.

There are thus two precursors to the tertiary process, dreams and pregenital problem solving, the former associated with the emergence of the primary process, the latter with that of the secondary and its partial integration with the primary. In the healthy case the tertiary process begins with invocations to solve problems that involve manageable levels of emotional intensity, the failure of which sees the child being overwhelmed with frustration over its limited problem solving powers but not of an order that can inhibit further growth. If the presenting problem is a frustrated wish whose resolution via a dream fails then the child wakes up with no implied limitation on subsequent growth.

Note again that dreams are an entirely intrapsychic event but that early or pregenital problem solving is usually, but not always, referred to an external object. The exception forms a connecting link for how the precursor becomes the tertiary process itself. Dream formation sees problem solving via imagery but without reality modifying action directed to the outer world, although some such action may take place intrapsychically. Pregenital problem solving begins to add both logic and some action to the formation of imagery that the secondary process regards as viable, usually but not always directed outward.

The tertiary process arises as the oedipal attachment takes place because the precursors must be jointly summoned to deal with a problem of unprecedented emotional intensity and risk. The tertiary process subsumes both dream formation and the use of logic and action for elementary problem solving associated with new and higher affective intensities that arise in the third stage. The defining characteristics of the tertiary process include a fuller integration of the primary and secondary processes and the ego strength for both processes and their integration to respond to problems with higher affective intensities; the results involve relations with objects outside the self, both personal and impersonal. Here the idea of ego strength is that alluded to earlier, the ability to summon all needed psychic parts in response to a challenge without fragmenting but rather with some likely prospects of success arising from the orchestration of the parts in the work of creating a proposed solution.

The work of nature to evolve the precursors up to the tertiary process implies certain changes for both the primary and secondary processes. Within the third stage the primary process is invoked with increasingly large numbers of attributes resulting in smaller numbers of candidate objects that can carry them. However, the intensity of the affective attributes rises considerably at this time and places a stronger demand on connecting emotional energy with the objects prior to their being winnowed down by the secondary process. The primary process enters and acquires within the third stage increasing capacity to manage mobile energy, this being a part of the configuration of the emerging tertiary process. The increased affective intensities or amounts of emotional energy carried by objects delivered by the primary to the secondary process place a greater demand on the latter's focusing function. At the same time maturation is increasing the number of attributes than can be used to define an object and hence a greater demand in the way of object discrimination arises. The tertiary process arises, in part, as something of a manager of the evolving primary and secondary processes. Its management role is subordinate to generating candidate solutions to presenting problems or challenges. As the role of the dream maker is to generate a scenario for the fulfilment of an internal wish, the role of the tertiary process is generate an actionable solution in response to the wish to solve a problem, where the action is usually external but could also be internal or mixed. As noted, the role of object relationships in the emergence of the tertiary process strongly distinguishes it from its precursors in the dream maker and pregenital problem solving.

Before dealing with the obvious fact that the tertiary process is another term for the creative mechanism or even dealing with a sharp definition of the mechanism, the role of the Oedipus complex in driving the unfolding of the tertiary process from its precursors needs to be examined more closely. Throughout the third stage the oedipal longing presents a child with increasingly strong emotional trends connected with a possessive love attachment to one parent with ever mounting fear of loss of love and some form of punishment by the other. The chronic frustration the child experiences eventually inclines the child to accept that its ambitious hopes cannot possibly be realized but before that happens the child's personality is engaged with the largest yet challenge of its life: how to win and also avoid punishment. Freud's explicit writing on the topic emphasized the affective or motivational aspects of the attachment but, as noted, his implicit writings recognize inner work on increasing the child's problem solving capacity. And more, he regards the then rising capacity to be a prototype for all subsequent pursuits of success, or problem solving to follow in the child's life.

Since it is in the nature of reality for all efforts to win the oedipal victory to include avoiding dire consequences, the tertiary process must make ever greater demands, in the sense of emotional load, on the primary and secondary processes. At the same time the child's ego strength for managing frustration, anxiety and repeated failure must rise to sustain the effort. The tertiary process uses the same kind of invocations of the primary and secondary processes as the dream maker but in the context of outside the self object relations and sustained frustration, the latter because renunciation is the only feasible solution to the problem. On the other hand, the wished for tertiary process outcome has to be a feasible way of solving the problem of winning the oedipal victory whereas for the dream maker the outcome is limited to a scenario. A part of the tertiary process must perform the work of studying the tentative objects delivered by its coordinated management of the primary and secondary processes for their role in a solution that can be tested for real world feasibility. The parallel work in dream formation is the review of the objects for a wish fulfilling role in a scenario that meets superego and reality constraints while preserving sleep. The Oedipus complex engages the precursors of dream formation and pregenital problem solving with drives that are both action and object related, building a mechanism that can do far more than solve the problem of creating a wish fulfilling dream scenario.

These considerations suggest why nature presents a child with the unsolvable problem of the Oedipus complex. Success in any part of life almost always requires repeated effort, with first efforts resulting in failure and frustration, followed by learning and modification of prior efforts, not to mention recovery of one's energy. The play work of children has some of these qualities but at very mild levels compared to what life after childhood will bring them. Managing frustration calls for ego strength but making repeated efforts calls for a perceived high value in what the undertaking is. A child entering the Oedipus complex has little, if any, awareness that what its drives are impelling it toward is impossible to achieve. A child tries many things to craft a winning oedipal strategy, not least among them studying the ways of the desired parent that please the rival parent with an eye for making the same kind of offerings in a better, that is more competitive, way. The endeavor, in the healthy case, sees the tertiary process responding to one invocation after another to arrive at a workable solution, all these part of the maturing the process itself. It also sees growth in the ability not just to sustain frustration but also to sustain hope.

That nature well knows what life after childhood will be like leads to the proposition that the Oedipus complex is intended by nature to lay down a prototype for all later problem solving, but with a proviso. Presenting the child with an impossible problem with emotional intensity of an entirely new order inducts the child into the needed modes of functioning that can solve the later problems of life. That is, the proviso is that while the child cannot find a solution to the oedipal problem, the resulting psychological gains prepare it to make efforts at problem solving that can succeed in later life. The unconscious equating of later attempts at success with oedipal victory generates ongoing hope and energy to sustain the effort. The impossibility of oedipal triumph results in a prototype for later efforts at success where success is feasible. Here the mechanistic part is the tertiary process but the energic, or motivational, part arises from equating current efforts with the first effort within the oedipal triangle. The dynamic involved is captured in many vulgarisms that equate strong interest in success in a given area with sexual excitement, such as saying of a person with a strong interest in creating success that he or she has an erection for it, although in less polite terms.

A part of the resulting third stage outcome or prototype is the same as the creative mechanism, a term that needs clarification. The adjective creative summons up images of fine art and other majestic works yet a child that learns to play a game is working in the same spirit because both kinds of endeavor begin with a wish to create a solution to a problem. In the first case the wish is along aesthetic lines and in the second it is more along the lines of creating mastery. Both involve invocations of the creative mechanism, although at widely different levels of challenge. The manner in which the tertiary process functions is the same whether a problem involves a great deal of invocation or very little. The first order of business for it is to determine if the presenting problem has already been solved, a thing that involves the use of memory. In the latter case the tertiary process still works to solve the problem, although the invocations of the primary and secondary processes may be minimal or null. This leads to the concept of perturbation in problem solving.

Given a problem to solve the tertiary process will first find a previously solved problem, if it exists, whose attributes most fully agree with those of the new problem based on the likelihood that a new solution will be a perturbation, or modification, of the old one. More precisely, a solution by perturbation is the result of making a small change to the known solution of another problem that has some resemblance to the new one and finding that it works. The basis for this is in invoking the primary and secondary processes with the sum of the attributes that belong to the new problem and the old one and proceeding as previously outlined. If no prior solution exists then the tertiary process will delete one or more attributes of the new problem and repeat the effort. Note here that perturbing prior solutions includes the use of pregenital ones formed by the precursors to the tertiary process, reflecting the cumulative nature of the problem solving mechanism. This adds to the motivation for regarding all forms of problem solving as instances of the use of the creative mechanism, however grand, nominal or trivial they are.

If all such efforts based on prior solutions fail then the principle of inheritance is applied. A class is formed all of whose objects carry at least one attribute of the problem at hand. The sum of all the attributes of all the objects in this class is formed, and then the secondary process is invoked to find objects that carry as many of the resulting set of attributes as possible. All such objects form candidates for inclusion in a solution scenario. If all such efforts fail then the problem is, pro temp, not solvable. The resulting set will tend to be very large because any one object need only carry one of the many attributes indicated. This begins to associate to the sense of desperation that often follows repeated failure in finding a solution, leading to the clutching at straws reaction often seen in states of panic.

Perturbing a known prior solution in search of a new one based on it has its roots in the fact that a problem and its solution must share attributes. More exactly the solution to a problem will carry some of the attributes of the problem it solves. For example, in dream formation the problem consists of things wished for and the solution is the hallucinatory presentation of them in the dream. As another example, a person seeking relief of emotional problems will seek a therapist who can relieve them and here some of the shared attributes are hope, where this refers to the patient's wish for relief and the therapist's wish to provide it, and emotional intelligence because the patient needs more of it and the therapist may provide it. When the tertiary process calls upon the primary and secondary processes it is using the inherent relationship between problem and solution attributes. There are pre-images of this in dream formation where the attributes of a wish are gathered and followed by the formation of classes of objects that carry those attributes. Within the creative mechanism aspect of the tertiary process the same procedure is followed but rather than a dream resulting, a solution scenario is created which is then reviewed by the secondary process for feasibility, the precursor for this being secondary revision in dream formation.

As an example of solving a new problem using a prior solution consider a clothing designer faced with the problem of doing something about the fact that people often outgrow their pants' size. This can be rephrased as what to do about the decrease in the comfort of how pants fit as the wearer puts on weight. There is no need to cite the attributes of the old problem of designing pants in the usual way because that is the solution to an old problem to be perturbed into a new solution for the current one. The attributes of the problem include growth, leg garment, comfort and goodness of fit where the last three attributes also belong to the definition of the old problem of designing pants. Some of the objects that carry all of these attributes include Bermuda shorts, swim suits, long johns, underwear, aquatic boots, pant suits and overalls. Note that all seven objects are made of either fabric or a variety of elastic and so accommodate growth to some degree. When this set of objects is reviewed by the secondary process the object underwear will stand out because it has the greatest capacity to accommodate growth via its elastic banding. When this is given to the overseeing tertiary process the union of pants and elastic banding leads to a visualization of their union, by methods not yet understood, and this results in an image of pants with some elastic banding to allow for stretch. This new solution is a perturbation of the old one. This solution by perturbation is much easier than one by inheritance, building as it does on the past, but it is likely to be less creative than what solution by inheritance can offer. Taking the liberty of Ignoring expense, a hypothetical solution by inheritance could result in a banding that uses pressure sensors in real time to compute how tight the banding ought to be for comfort, followed by microprocessor adjustment of the tension in the banding, where the banding consists of vertical filaments of adjustable magnetic strength enabling both attraction and repulsion and with a battery as a power source embedded in the belt.

The tertiary process as a high order ego function must have access to many different ancillary ego functions such as logic, imaging, calculating, processing sensory feedback and so on. These are cited to allude to the complexity of the work done by the process, the present goal being to outline its overall structure. The inner knowing of the tertiary process that problems and their solutions share attributes is expressed in the use of reverse engineering which begins with a solution, understood as a device, and works backward to its design principles, these reflecting the problem it solves. This is seen very clearly in science fiction where an alien craft is examined to divine its principles of operation and hence the problems they solve.

The tertiary process includes more than the creative mechanism. Unlike one of its precursors, the dream mechanism that creates a scenario which is then played before the remains of consciousness in sleep, the work of the creative mechanism is a candidate for action, usually externally directed. As the dream mechanism must be connected to ego powers that display the scenario, the tertiary process must have access to motor activity that expresses the actions in the recommended solution. There is recursion in dream formation because of repeated efforts to find objects that sufficiently meet requirements as well as in evaluations of proposed scenarios formed with the given objects. Similarly within the tertiary process the recommended action must be studied for success as a thought experiment, not yet performed in reality.[31] However once a solution is regarded as testable in reality it must be carried out and if not sufficiently successful a fresh recommended solution must be generated, this being a form of recursion not seen in dream formation because dreams build to scenarios and not to reality modifying actions. The next effort at a solution will include attributes acquired from the experiment with the first solution. These considerations further support regarding all forms of problem solving as instances of the use of the creative mechanism. That intellectual problem solving, as seen in mathematics and the hard sciences, is included within the tertiary process only means that little, if any motor action, is expended after a proposed solution is formed.

Many things can go awry, both with respect to motivation and mechanism, within the formation of the tertiary process, this forming the subject matter of the next chapter.

---

[31] Recall here Freud's view that thought is a form of experimental action involving small displacements of energy.

CHAPTER 7

HEALING, GROWTH AND THE TERTIARY
PROCESS

Freud felt that the third stage witnessed two pivotal events. The first is the achievement of a foundational form for all later development of the personality, a corollary of which is that no significant psychopathology can be created after the ending of this stage. The second event, which he regarded as integral to the unfolding of this final form, both in terms of motivation and mechanism, is the Oedipus complex. His lifelong goal was to contribute to an understanding of nature with the hope of relieving human suffering and, latterly, with the hope of improving both adaptation and culture. His focus on the relationship between emotional health and the ability to create success in life increased as his insights into pathology deepened. This is strongly correlated with his emphasis on the Oedipus complex as the central and final event of childhood in the formation of the personality and its preparation to adapt to all later events in life. It is also correlated with his view that every analysis builds to resolving that complex.

His summary definition of health is that a person is healthy if that person can work and love, it being implicit that performance in either area is sufficient to result in satisfaction. As for achieving such a state of health his position was that the major goals of an analysis are to well enough resolve both the Oedipus complex and latent homosexuality, where well enough means that any residual pathology can no longer significantly interfere with adaptation and an acceptable quality of life. The matter of latent homosexuality enters because Freud's model regards human nature as inherently bisexual and hence a failure to live the homosexual aspect can only result in pathology and limitations; the underlying assumption here is that both trends of sexuality are crafted by nature to serve adaptation.

The adaptive limitations, and also suffering, of a person who is mostly hysterical are rooted in the way the person's Oedipus complex comes to end, it being implicit that the outcomes of the oral and anal stages have been sufficient to support genital stage unfolding. For Freud the Oedipus complex was a beautiful but ill fated drama whose working through called upon all prior developments. Its central theme is ambitious love whose outcome has much to do with creating and failing to create success in life. In the simplest theoretical case an hysteric is developmentally arrested only in the genital stage as a result of unmanageable stresses within the Oedipus complex. The stresses can have many forms including parental anxiety over the child's wishes, a childishly competitive attitude in the rival parent or such things as the wished for parent turning to the child's oedipal attachment for satisfactions that are compensatory for frustrations with the rival parent. In all instances the defining, but not the only, defense used is repression to keep the oedipal attachment and its associated stresses away from consciousness. The stresses, together with fear of punishment, led Freud to the formulation that the superego is heir to the Oedipus complex. This is a motivational statement and not a mechanistic one. The superego legacy of the Oedipus complex for most children is both fear of success and limited capacity to create it, these being motivational and mechanistic respectively.

The motivational deficit is seen in the composition of some of the primary process's equivalence classes. Note that the fact that the process has a well formed structure for forming equivalence classes does not necessarily imply that all its classes are well formed, this being a distinction between a container and what is contained. This is seen, for example, in primary process classes that represent the issues of fear of success and guilt over creating it. That these two issues are related but not identical is seen in the different ways in which some of their corresponding classes are formed. Since the tertiary process, as well as the creative mechanism, are formed with the unfolding of the Oedipus complex, and since this complex becomes an unconscious prototype for later pursuits of success, it follows that the child's regard for success in later life features the same or similar affective responses as in the original pursuit. Fear of punishment, castration in the male, evisceration in the female, are major factors ending this first pursuit of success. Putting to one side, for the moment, that reality eventually inclines the child to give up the pursuit, these punishments become connected with later strivings for success. The outcome can only be limited tertiary response in generating testable solutions to the problem of how to create success in any one instance. The objects in primary process classes that carry the attributes of success will now also carry fearful, even dreaded, attributes limiting the workings of the tertiary process that invokes it. The power of the secondary process to discriminate between what is to be feared versus not will have limited capacity to do so when it comes to objects needed for success. Indeed, the tertiary process at the very outset of the wish to create success will have blunted capacity to invoke both the primary and secondary processes, the connection of strong anxiety with the idea of success looming over the idea itself. The workings of the creative mechanism as a tertiary process coordination of primary and secondary process invocations is limited as a consequence of all three issues.

The matter of guilt over creating success as an oedipal outcome limits tertiary process unfolding in ways similar to those seen in fear of success and therefore the nature of healing and growth within resolving hysteria with respect to both guilt and fear may be treated simultaneously. There are a number of equivalence class malformations within the primary process that need healing in order for growth to take place. In the case of a male, for example, the mother's attributes will include anxiety, guilt, risk and danger. In the case of ideal health the attributes anxiety and guilt would only be present at low levels of affective intensity; the attributes of risk and danger would not be present at all, except in possibly transient situations such as a bout of ill health in the mother. Anxiety is present because of fear of punishment by the father as well as well as of the presence of guilt; guilt is present for fear of losing the father's love and as a reaction to resentment for the father as a rival; risk also enters as an associate of both castration anxiety and guilt. This describes elements of incorrect attributions of the mother as an object that propagate into the primary process construction of equivalence classes, these being malformations.

Propagation takes place via inheritance in which the primary process assigns attributes of one member of a class to some or all of the other members. This is an instance of displacement, as seen in dream and symptom formation, but its use in developmentally arrested parts of the personality where the tertiary process is too poorly formed to invoke secondary process correction, leads to object representations that are, in some way, simply unrealistic. In the above example, the propagation of the mother as an anxiety figure results in the given person unconsciously perceiving females in general as anxiety provoking, whether this refers to fear of success or to guilt or both. Incorrect representations of objects can only lead to frequent instances of poor adaptation, a familiar companion of neurosis, whether hysteria or worse because of insufficient perception of reality and false attributions.

In hysteria the emotional force that prevents the secondary process from correcting such inheritances is mostly the defense of repression. In the case of a male the work of defense is to keep the child unaware of its father dread, which leads to anxiety in relation to the mother, and limits the capacity of the tertiary process to use the secondary to study and correct the attributions of the primary, as noted. The general treatment goal is to enable the subject to deal with oedipal stresses in a more adult or evolved way than via the avoidance methods of defense. Evidence of such healing and growth is found in more mature actions of the tertiary process, as observable in the corrections of malformed classes of objects. The lifting of repression enables coordinated use of the secondary process to review such malformations as they surface within therapeutically driven anxiety arsing from transference. The work of interpretation enables the secondary process to see the lack of correspondence with reality in relevant primary process classes that are evoked by it. Evidence that working through is taking place is seen in increasingly appropriate affective responses which, in turn, reflect correction of object representations within the classes that any one interpretation touches upon. The healing aspect of this is the deletion of attributes that do not realistically belong to a given object; the growth aspect is the addition of attributes that do in fact describe the given objects.

Some deletions will be the full removal of an attribute and some will be changes in its intensity, so that some of the original attribution is retained as a qualitative tag while the intensity or degree of its presence is the locus of change. Note that all three modifications – deleting attributes, changing their intensity or adding new ones – are movements of primary process toward secondary functioning with respect to object representations. It can happen that the starting representation remains within a primary process class even though the new representation has been formed. The sense of this is that the starting representation may be needed for creative work whereas the latter is needed more in assessing the candidate objects produced by the primary process in working on subsequent problems. Such assessment is weak in dream formation but far more vigorous in problem solving. All this points to reduced reliance on primary process functioning and increased reliance on secondary process functioning as treatment outcomes.

Such local evidence of healing and growth within the primary and secondary processes is also evidence of systemic change in the way the subject is dealing with oedipal stresses that damaged the personality, this being more evolved tertiary process functioning. For example, the attribution of risk, anxiety or danger to the mother as propagated to all females will either be deleted or reduced in intensity in some, possibly all, classes. Similarly, dread of the father as propagated to males similar to the father in key ways will undergo like changes.

Successful analysis should result in increased frustration tolerance in the hysterical subject. This revisits the problem of the oedipal goal being entirely unachievable, no matter how many attempts at success are made. This seems to imply that the attribute of frustration will propagate to all objects involved in the later pursuits of success because the prototype for success is infeasible, and therefore will limit, or even inhibit, all such later efforts. It is at this point that Freud's view of the superego as the heir to the Oedipus complex enters. The dread of punishment is a strong factor in bringing the attachment to a close and inclining the child to accept the impossibility of its ambitions. However the superego formations that result are not only prohibitive but also define allowable means of oedipal like satisfaction with non-family members. When this option is combined with the use of sublimation many other avenues of satisfaction open to the child and a more endorsing part of the superego is also formed. The tertiary process revisits the many attributions of frustration that arose within the complex and lowers their intensities for objects that are deemed allowable. This adds to what growth in frustration tolerance took place and supports tertiary process engagement of the primary and secondary process in problem solving. That is, excessive frustration levels as inhibiting factors are undone resulting in objects needed for success formulations to be identified. The comparative presence of low versus high attributions of frustration indicates the degree of success or failure in healing and growth.

Another outcome of the oedipal triangle is the establishment of a stereotypy within the hysteric. It is a neurotic part of self identity that arises to compensate for the inevitable acceptance of the child's ambition as being unachievable. This acceptance is a blow to self esteem as well as to motivation to pursue success elsewhere. The child, sensing its already existing strengths as well as society's success stereotypes soon also senses that some among the latter accommodate those strengths. The blow to oedipal ambition is mitigated by the adoption of a stereotype that the child feels it can live and thereby increases its feeling that success is possible; the word 'increases' enters because the oedipal outcome, as already noted, does result in a reduction of the drive and capacity to create that initial success. However, the stronger that blow, the greater the need for a stereotypy to compensate. A common stereotypy among men is that of Don Juan and among women is that of a femme fatale, both leading to repeated assurance that one can win in love. These stereotypies also lead to over-focus on winning in love and to under-focus on many other areas of life where success can be created. Some other common stereotypies are the savvy businessman, the saint, the leader, the savant, the warrior and so on.

A sign of healing and growth in an hysteric would be changes in the object representations of things needed for success outside the stereotypy. Attributes such as hope and satisfaction would be added to such objects and those allied with anxiety would either be dropped or diminished in intensity. Both such changes increase secondary process functioning and decrease primary process functioning. It may happen that a given object loses an attribute and gains none, this appearing at first to make its representation more primary process like but if the result more faithfully represents reality with fewer attributes then this is in the spirit of the secondary process. Another sign would be an increase in the capacity of the tertiary process to marshal more intense affects for connection with candidate objects, and a corresponding gain in the amount of affect the secondary process can focus in formulating a proposed solution. A decrease in flooding, a prominent symptom of hysteria, would also be seen in this increased power of focus

Outgrowing hysterical fantasies with more courting of reality is related to the decrease in flooding that follows the weakening of repressions. Such fantasies serve essentially the same purpose as a stereotypy in providing alternate means of satisfaction, although the latter provides more of a sense of capacity to create success. With both of these the tertiary process is ever vigilant of the nature of reality in its role as a problem solving mechanism. As the repressions that led to both are undone the tertiary process becomes more enabled to solve the problem of both fantasies and stereotypies limiting problem solving ability itself, this in conjunction with pursuit of success. The tertiary process locates objects that enter fantasies to create the appearance of satisfaction from an illusory gain and removes or diminishes the intensity of attributes that lead to the illusion. The resulting objects become less primary process like and more secondary process like as a result of these actions. The parallel changes that result from undoing a stereotypy are the undoing, in objects, of attributes that oppose success and the addition of such ones as feasibility, ambition and hope to success related objects..

With obsessionals the tertiary process has less to build on or to emerge from and is consequently less completely formed than with an hysteric. Developmental arrest within the anal stage implies a general rigidity of personality to one degree or another depending on how early in the anal stage it occurs. Such rigidity limits the interface between the primary process and the secondary because the former, assuming it to be well formed, can allocate large amounts of affect but the latter is only partially able to manage them. One outcome of this is that the secondary process emerges with limited capacity to assign affective attributes to objects. At the same time the secondary process, because of its growth in reality sense and its rigidly favoring cognitive over affective attributes, will tend to assign many attributes to an object, but with few of them being affective. That is, the reality sense develops strongly in the area of objects that carry little feeling and weakly otherwise and the ability to perceive small non-emotional differences between objects is pronounced. The general affective rigidity also implies that the propagation of attributes via inheritance is limited, an outcome that affects many processes. Among them are creativity and problem solving in the emotional area, the interpretation of the emotional content of events, formulation of ideas that are emotionally charged and empathic response in many areas.

The rigidity is mostly an outcome of a strong reaction formation against aggressive trends such as rage, hate and anger, these three being related but distinct in meaning. This results in the associated attributes being assigned to many more objects than reality supports. Long associative chains can result in absurdities such as dread of blocked rage becoming experienced as dread of clowns or buildings with the thirteenth floor missing. Such chains would be formed via the primary process, assumed mostly intact, but the strong lack of connection with aspects of reality would be exaggerated by the shortfalls in the secondary process.

One result of these considerations is that the tertiary process emerges with less capacity to coordinate the primary and secondary processes than in hysteria. This is often easy to see when an obsessional tries to resolve an emotional problem with labored thinking when more feeling contact is needed, the outcome often being a foggy state or abulia.

One of the main therapeutic goals is to weaken the defense of reaction formation against blocked rage to enable the subject to slowly become more able to experience emotional and feeling processes. An associated goal is the undoing of the same defense, as well as secondary ones such as denial and repression, to gain access to unconscious guilt because the guilt is reactive to the blocked rage. The melting of rigidity and the onset of increased emotional experience and expression are easy to observe qualitative changes. Less easy to observe is increased problem solving ability. Progress in achieving these goals is seen in well defined changes in all three processes, primary, secondary and tertiary.

One sign of the weakening of rigidity in an obsessional is the assignment of more affective attributes to object representations as well as the connection of higher levels of affect with objects selected by the primary process for membership in a given class. This is also a sign of increased lability. A corresponding gain in tertiary process functioning is the capacity for such objects, when reviewed by the secondary process, to focus higher levels of affect in the formulation of tentative solutions, whether for dreams or problem solving. The downgrading of unconscious guilt will result in lower intensities of that affect in the representations of objects that are or can be pleasing to the subject. The implied rise in self esteem sees increased intensities of positive affective attributes and the addition of more such to the representation of the self. Increases in frustration tolerance as a result of successful interpretive work are seen in decreases of negative affects of objects that carry such attributes as ambition and success.

The corresponding gains in ego strength, understood as the capacity to summon all needed capacities to meet a challenge, are seen in increasing numbers of attributes used to define objects. The larger such numbers are, the larger the number of associated classes defined by subsets of them as created by invocations of the primary process under the tertiary in solution formulation, all this needing a 'holding together' of tentative results by the latter process. The first kind of increase, in numbers of attributes used to define objects, may be temporary as with real time problem solving, or enduring as in object representations laid down in memory, the latter also being a result of increased reality testing as a treatment outcome.

The fact that the defining symptoms of the disorder, obsessing and compulsing, load on thinking and acting, reveals where to look for signs of their abatement. Obsessing is a defensive way of avoiding strong feelings, usually rage, that are regarded as dangerous to or unmanageable for consciousness. The act of obsessing features visit after visit to the same idea, a thing seen in ever more attributes being added to the current representation of the objects involved. This is a form of action that results in consuming some of the emotional energy of the blocked affects, an emotionally costly and usually painful way to deal with the given affects. As the trend to obsess diminishes the accumulation of ever more attributes, in real time and possibly in memory, occurs less and less frequently. This also leads to less stalling of the tertiary process, and hence increased availability of the process to deal with non-neurotic or real problems, because of the abatement of the fixedness of attention within obsessing. The increased availability refers both to invoking the creative mechanism for recommended solutions as well as the carrying out and testing of those solutions, this involving the tertiary process's access to motor activity.

As obsessing fixes on thought to avoid affective experience, compulsing fixes on action to achieve the same end. For reasons rooted in the individual history of associations and experiences in any one instance, an action takes on an anxiety reducing meaning. To cite a common literary example, compulsive cleaning is often a way to relieve unconscious guilt; compulsively putting things in order is often a way to create an unconscious sense of certainty that one's blocked rage is securely blocked or under control. The given behavior involves a displacement of unmanageable emotional intensity and/or meaning onto a task that consciousness can manage via certain actions such as rituals or avoidances. This means that certain attributes have been inappropriately added to the inner representation of the objects involved and hence healing and growth would see a decrease in their intensity or their removal. Inappropriate additions reflect weakness in the power of the tertiary process to manage the interface between the primary and secondary processes. Compulsing as a means of managing overly strong unconscious trends is both inefficient and a sign of under developed reality sense. The tertiary process in carrying out such actions fails to see these things, this reflecting again poor management of the cited interface. Healing and growth here involve primary and secondary process improvements and hence also increases in reality sense.

The borderline disorder is regarded as being on the boundary between neurosis and psychosis because borderlines, under nominal conditions, adapt mostly as a neurotic would but under sufficient stress begin to adapt psychotically. Splitting is a defining defense and refers to the lack of integration of the subject's representations of the perceived good and bad parts of another person or object. It indicates some degree of oral fixation and it is therefore not surprising that merging is also a major defense with a borderline, the defense raising the subject's sense of inner wellness by regarding the strength of another as being in the self; this involves melting of boundaries. The low ego strength in borderlines is often seen in inability to hold a job or remain committed to a task, life events that tend to invoke merging as a compensation. Frustration tolerance is low because splitting leads to seeing another as all good or all bad, the former leading to merging, the latter to rejection of the other. Splitting, merging and low frustration tolerance, taken together makes long term, satisfying work and relationships unlikely.

It is characteristic of splitting for the subject to have separated representations of the good and bad attributes of a given person or object. One sign of healing and growth with respect to splitting would be the formation of a third representation which, as a treatment outcome, draws the attributes of the separated classes to itself, giving rise to a more integrated representation of the given object. Within this the separated representations would persist for as long as the subject's ego strength is low enough to require the defense of splitting, but with healing and growth these would tend to dissolve as the third representation is formed.

One sign of healing and growth with respect to merging is a slowing of the experience of the attributes of the other as belonging to the self. Since such an experience would propagate via inheritance to other objects in the class of the self, it follows that a sign of slowing would be a decrease in both the number of attributes of the other taken to belong to the self as well as in their number propagated via inheritance. In addition, since an increase in attributes implies more classes, whose membership rule is possessing some of those attributes, a sign of healing and growth would be a decrease in the number of classes overall. A conspicuous sign of healing of growth would be a decrease in the number of attributes used in the representation of the self.

The event of merging means that the attributes of another are regarded as attributes of the self, an event that can only take place with the suspension of the secondary process. A sign of healing and growth in merging would be the increasing capacity of the tertiary process to prevent the suspension, thus thwarting the accretion of the other's attributes to the self.

The low ego strength in a borderline is seen in many primary process equivalence classes being defined with small numbers of attributes, this resulting in low powers of discrimination. This, combined with the lack of integration of the subject's representations of another's good and bad parts often leads to poor reality testing of a kind usually seen in the psychoses. Evidence of successful treatment would be a greater use of classes defined by comparatively greater numbers of attributes, this also resulting in increased reality testing. This is also evidence of increased tertiary process capacity to coordinate the results of primary and secondary processes on the way to creating proposed solutions to life challenges or problems.

The borderline's low frustration tolerance results in limited unfolding of the action aspect of the tertiary process because of the limited ability to do the sustained work required to carry out recommended solutions and to reality test them, this being a part of convergence to a feasible solution. In many instances the problem solving part of the tertiary process is little past the workings of the dream mechanism and pregenital problem solving. The qualitative signs of healing and growth in this area that are easy to see in expressed emotion are also seen in changes in object representations. The attribution of duress or negative affect to objects declines as frustration tolerance increases with a resulting decrease in the size of classes whose definitions include such attributes. Similarly, the sizes of classes whose definition includes positive affective attributes such as satisfaction and perseverance increase.

Depressive psychosis announces itself loudly with such things as end of the world hallucinations and frequent merging, the former expressing the profound sense of emptiness in this disorder and the latter the desperate efforts to fill the self with life. The underlying cause is insufficient internalization of the mother or caring figure(s), this resulting in large shortfalls in the creation of the good object. There is frequent raging against the self often resulting in hallucinations of parents, or their equivalent, this being a psychotic defense against superego pressure based on putting the creators of the superego back outside the self where they originated. This is a primitive primary process event in which elements of what are inside come to belong to the class of things outside. This level of pathology is driven not so much by regressive retreat from the Oedipus complex as in failures in the caring function in the oral stage, although there may be regression from the anal stage.

Although Freud felt there was little hope for successful treatment of psychotics, because of their minimal capacity for transference, his following eventually found a technique that promises some success. A major part of the therapeutic strategy with neurotics is to frustrate the patient's infantile wishes within the transference because satisfying them does not result in healing and growth but rather repetition of the wishes. However it was eventually discovered that satisfying some infantile wishes with psychotics, such as being mothered, can result in healing and growth. Very likely the brain mechanisms within psychotics are so arrested that the infant's ability to grow in response to emotional cues is still in place, a thing entirely untrue of neurotics.

The level of maturity of the tertiary process within depressive psychosis is mostly limited to the dream mechanism and pregenital problem solving. The comments on merging given for the borderline apply here also, but to a much greater degree because of the profound sense of emptiness. The incompleteness or near absence of the good object results in many classes either lacking sufficient positive attributes and/or having, inappropriately, many negative or hurtful ones, the latter reflecting not just the sense of emptiness but also the presence of a raging superego, punishing the self for not being good enough to obtain more loving care.

Evidence of healing and growth is not seen so much in the tertiary process as in abatement of merging, as with the borderline, and of the use of hallucinations and delusions and some lifting of mood. Hallucinations, like merging have to do with self versus non-self discrimination. In order for an inner image to appear to be in the class of things outside the self – assuming a bodily hallucination is not referred to – the attributes associated with it, although giving it outside the self class membership, must also pass whatever level of secondary process functioning is present. Since the inner image precursor to an hallucination begins as a part of the self, the secondary process must fail to see this and therefore healing and growth in this area imply that either this capacity is restored, if lost regressively, or created in the first place otherwise. In the sequel the hallucination loses membership in the class of things outside the self and a gain in secondary process representation results. Since the tertiary process emerges after the primary and secondary processes, improvements in the latter are likely to enable improvements in the former, making some further evolution of the tertiary process expectable, but not to any large degree. If a bodily hallucination, such as worms crawling on one's skin, is referred to, the attribute of self must be among those of the precursor (worms) and a similar secondary process failure occurs with similar remarks on healing and growth.

A delusion is not as primitive a symptom as an hallucination, but in parallel with it, a delusion begins with a precursor idea that the subject wants to be true of reality. The delusion must be made to belong to the class of things regarded as real or valid and this requires that the secondary process be unable to see the contradictions between the attributes of the precursor and those of the object whose meaning is being distorted. Healing and growth here imply the restoration of the secondary process, or if not yet created, its creation, followed by the removal of the attribute of reality from the object representations connected with the delusion. This in turn results in one or more primary process classes moving toward a more secondary process character, with mild tertiary process gains as with hallucinations..

Healing and growth with respect to mood should lead to some increase in the size or presence of the good object and less turning of rage upon the self. Increasing presence of the good object leads to less pessimism and negative expectation in addition to some improvement in mood. The number of objects in classes that carry such attributes as pessimism or negative expectations would thus decrease and the number of objects in classes carrying such attributes as hope or positive expectation would increase. Mood improvement would lead to a decrease in the number of negative attributes in the representation of the self and an increase in the number of positive ones. Such changes would propagate via inheritance to objects in classes to which the self, as an object, belongs. Such inheritance would be realistic where the secondary process well functions and otherwise would not.

Such gains would naturally lead to evolution in the tertiary process as a problem solver, but more to the point, also to gains in the capacity of the process to engage the personality to carry out proposed solutions. As a corollary increases in frustration tolerance are expectable with a fall off of negative attributions in the definitions both of classes and objects belonging to classes.

Schizophrenia is a good example of Freud's summary that in psychosis, the unconscious is conscious. One example of this is hallucinating, shared with depressive psychosis, because it is a waking dream or, equivalently, a dream is a hallucination during sleep. The disturbance of language seen in schizophrenia is another example because a schizophrenic word construction tends to be a primary process precursor of what results, in healthier people, in cogent sentences via secondary process review. Far and away the defining sign of a schizophrenic is fragmentation of personality, as if it came forward in fits and starts with little integration. The schizophrenic use of language illustrates this because of the lack of tertiary process coordination of the primary process with what level of secondary process capacity has been achieved. An easily observable consequence of fragmentation is a profound level of infantilism and poor ego strength. Many of their adaptations take place at a primary process level of understanding of reality where objects belonging to the same class take each other's place in dealing with reality. The level of maturation of the tertiary process is little past the dream mechanism and pregenital problem solving, as with depressive psychotics but with the difference that schizophrenics are developmentally arrested earlier in the oral stage than the latter.

Given the profound level of arrest in this disorder, signs of healing and growth are found mostly in maturation of the primary process with movement toward secondary process functioning. A distinguishing sign of psychosis versus neurosis is the disturbance in the relation to reality that characterizes the former. Hence the class defined by the attribute of being real contains many unrealistically represented objects some of which will be delusions and hallucinations. A sign of healing and growth here would be an increase in the number of classes defined by more than previously used numbers of attributes and a decrease in the number of classes defined by small numbers, this indicating an increase in differentiation along with increased reality sense.

Signs of progress in resolving fragmentation are found in a reduction in the number of parts of the self unconsciously perceived as separated, a result of a degree of integration leading to two or more parts becoming joined as a part of a larger whole that subsumes each of them. The clinical sign of this quantitative change would be a reduction in organismic panic, or the intense fear of coming apart into separated pieces. Since much of the disorder is based on inadequate self versus non self differentiation, improvement would be seen in a decrease of the number of objects that belong to the class defined by the self, this also being a secondary process gain. The last gain indicates an improvement in the tertiary process because of the implied increase in the ability of the secondary process to review and evaluate primary process objects recommended as parts of a solution to a problem. A decrease in fragmentation implies an improvement in the tertiary process's capacity to act on its recommended solutions to problems, and this, two taken with the prior gain, indicates overall improvement in this process. +

Paranoia is regarded as a subtype of schizophrenia. The pervasive symptom of suspicion with delusions of persecution correlate well with a common sense idea of psychosis, but paranoia's relation to fragmenting is not as apparent. Freud's formulation of blocked homosexual trends as fundamental in causing paranoia is a key to making sense of this.

In the case of a male a typical event sequence leading to paranoia begins with castration anxiety within the oedipal attachment to the mother strong enough to drive a regression away from her to earlier forms of love for her. It is assumed that this takes place in the context of insufficient anal developments that enable the regression to continue back to the oral stage, while also keeping some anal powers intact. The heterosexual love of the oedipal attachment is renounced and replaced by the earlier, pre-oedipal, love for the mother within which the child identifies with her. The child uses its identification with the mother to assume those of her ways that please the father to reduce castration anxiety, this becoming a homosexual orientation as the regression is sustained. The outcome for the paranoid-to-be is immense dread of castration anxiety in association with his homosexual longings based on the wish to be like his mother. The mechanism of paranoia is based on fear of a part of the self being seen. When the subject feels an unconscious homosexual interest in someone, the idea that females seduce men is triggered, leading to dread of castration because females do not have male genitals. This strong anxiety is consciously experienced in the derivative form of hurtful intentions on the part of the other who is homosexually desired.

The mechanism in the case of the female cannot be the same for obvious anatomical differences, however objectionable homosexual trends are also at the root of paranoia in the female. One proposed explanation is that the female, experiencing oedipal defeat, including possible lack of interest from the father or outright rejection by him, suffers a narcissistic wound the female child is unprepared to deal with because of inadequate maturation in the prior sexual stages. Here regression follows, as with the male, but for the female the regression is back to the earlier homosexual attachment to the mother reinforced by flight from the father. This accounts for the often seen contempt of men in lesbians. Another proposed explanation is that evisceration anxiety in females plays the role of castration anxiety in males, driving a fearful abandonment of the oedipal attachment with regression back to the mother, even though she would be the eviscerating figure. The sense of this is that abandoning the quest for the father ends (perceived) hostile rivalry with the mother in full analogy with the male child.

The fact that both genders are said to have unshakeable beliefs in their delusions of persecution is a key to understanding the connection between paranoia and fragmentation. However, outside their delusions much of their reality sense is not just intact but often highly evolved. One sign of this is that paranoids usually have considerable ability to mime normal behavior within their own culture, enabling them to hide their delusions. Their powers of observation and perception are usually overdeveloped in their vigilant search for potential persecutors. Unfortunately these highly developed powers are widely separated from their delusions because the latter protect them from seeing their unconscious homosexual trends. The wide separation is motivated by castration anxiety in the male and in either unbearable narcissistic injury or evisceration anxiety in the female. The presence of unshakeable beliefs in their delusions reflects the intensity of their underlying anxiety. As a result anyone who stirs homosexual longings in them is unconsciously seen as bringing them closer to their dreaded punishments and is therefore experienced as a persecutor.

The delusions are not only formed around individuals but also around groups and society, especially when these can serve defensive purposes. For example, it is common for paranoids to delusionally identify with the military because it represents power and hence denies castration, the delusion being that of an ordained leader or deliverer. This is clear in the case of a male paranoid but with a female the dynamics are more subtle. Renouncing the father as the oedipal object followed by moving it to the mother results in the child feeling that she no longer needs her father because her homosexual mother attachment makes her a male, in that it repeats the father's relation to the mother. At this point the longing for power that is transparent in the male child becomes apparent in the female. The dynamic has the as if quality of not needing the father because the female has become a male herself, a frequent behavior in lesbians.

It is also common for paranoids to have delusions regarding their government because, in reality, it has lawful powers of inspection and observation. These are taken delusionally to be the government out to hurt the paranoid with key knowledge of his or her life.

The wide separation between the paranoid's reality testing powers and his or her delusions is a first example of fragmentation. This occurs within an otherwise fragile ego with considerable oral and anal arrest. A number of overly strong stresses can collapse a paranoid's defenses, usually based on projection of the paranoid's hostility onto the longed for person, and result in fragmentation. One such stress is spontaneous biological change that increases libido, as often seen in change of life, for both genders. Another is too much repudiation of the paranoid's delusions, as can happen with public figures who draw much media criticism. Another, more familiar stress, is a paranoid being betrayed by a trusted follower or believer in his or her delusions. Such stresses rupture the defensive distance between reality testing powers and the dreaded impulses and make necessary more primitive defenses to keep those powers away from conscious experience. A primitive defense of choice is dedifferentiation in which inner structures and their relatedness to one another are undone in the desperate attempt to keep conscious perception away from the dreaded trends. The defense works by undoing the inner organization that can support the given perception, a truly pyrrhic victory. This is the very event of fragmentation.

Given the massive rigidity in paranoids, healing and growth is unlikely, though theoretically possible. There is little prospect of making the homosexual root of the disorder amenable to awareness but there can be some prospect of taming their immense suspicion. The strong presence of suspicion in paranoia means that any class whose defining attributes include suspicion or danger will be inappropriately large as a result of attributes of their delusions propagating, via inheritance, to other objects. A sign of healing would be a decrease in such numbers, this being an apparent move toward more primary process functioning. However, as such negative attributes are removed, where they do not in fact properly belong, the subject becomes more able to see the given objects as they are and this tends to result in a net increase in the number of attributes associated with them, and this is a movement toward increased secondary process functioning. Such gains imply an increase in the problem solving role of the tertiary process and, since there is a fall off in fear of others, the inclination to take action to test solutions to problems also rises, resulting in a gain in the tertiary process capacity to test solutions in reality.

If any progress is made in dealing with the homosexual root of paranoia then a number of changes in the representation of the self are expectable. In the case of a male, the idea of the self that has access to consciousness will come to acquire more feminine attributes and less victim ones because the unconscious dread of feminine trends has been lifted, to some degree. The situation with a female is parallel to this with dreaded masculine trends being replaced by feminine ones. Any progress at this level predicts for a prior undoing of some of the power of the delusions and therefore delusional attributes of the self would diminish. Examples of such delusions include the self as a savior, a sacrifice, a hero, a victim or prey. Evidence of increased self versus non self discrimination is much the same as with depressive psychosis, with the exception that this deficiency is more widespread in schizophrenia.

BIBLIOGRAPHY

Arieti, Silvano. 1976. *Creativity The Magic Synthesis*. New York: Basic Books.

Freud, Sigmund. 2001. *The Standard Edition of the Complete Psychological works of Sigmund Freud*. London: Vintage Books.

Jones, Ernest. 1961. *The Life and Works of Sigmund Freud*. New York: Basic Books.

Klein, Melanie. 1975. *Envy and Gratitude*. The Melanie Klein Trust: Delacorte Press.

Krohn, Alan. 1978. *Hysteria: The Elusive Disorder*. New York: International Universities Press.

Spitz, Rene. 1965. *The First Year of Life*. New York: International Universities Press.

INDEX

abreaction, 17, 19, 20

adaptation, ix, x, xi, 20, 29, 30, 67, 68, 69, 74, 77, 78, 82, 98, 100, 111, 113

aggression, 11, 25, 26, 27, 28, 70, 71, 73

ambition, 11, 93, 95, 115, 116, 118

anal sadistic, 25, 29

anxiety, ix, x, 2, 4, 5, 6, 7, 8, 13, 19, 22, 23, 24, 25, 26, 29, 33, 51, 52, 53, 58, 74, 75, 81, 92, 93, 95, 96, 101, 105, 112, 113, 114, 116, 118, 124, 125

Aristotle, 13, 48, 52, 55, 60

arrest, ix, 3, 19, 20, 26, 30, 32, 85, 116, 123, 126

association, 6, 8, 15, 16, 35, 42, 48, 64, 71, 72, 124

attribute, 53, 55, 57, 59, 60, 61, 65, 76, 77, 79, 82, 83, 84, 85, 93, 108, 114, 115, 116, 122, 123

attributes, 53, 54, 55, 56, 57, 58, 59, 60, 61, 62, 64, 67, 69, 70, 71, 72, 73, 74, 75, 76, 77, 79, 81, 82, 83, 84, 85, 86, 101, 102, 104, 107, 108, 109, 110, 112, 113, 114, 116, 117, 118, 119, 120, 121, 122, 123, 126, 127

bad object, 35, 36

borderline, ix, 36, 85, 119, 120, 121

castration, 22, 26, 33, 92, 93, 95, 112, 113, 124, 125

cathartic method, 15, 17

cathexis, 41, 44, 49, 68

censorship, 16

class, 29, 56, 57, 58, 59, 60, 62, 64, 65, 67, 70, 71, 72, 73, 75, 76, 77, 79, 83, 84, 85, 86, 93, 108, 113, 114, 117, 120, 121, 122, 123, 124, 126

classes, 32, 56, 59, 60, 64, 65, 67, 69, 71, 72, 73, 74, 75, 76, 77, 79, 85, 86, 101, 108, 112, 113, 114, 118, 119, 120, 121, 122, 123

component, vii, xi, 21, 24, 25, 29, 83, 87, 89, 91, 92

condensation, 56, 58, 59, 60, 62

dedifferentiation, 19, 33, 78, 86, 126

defense, ix, 2, 19, 20, 23, 24, 26, 27, 28, 30, 36, 41, 43, 63, 84, 85, 86, 112, 113, 117, 119, 120, 121, 126

delusion, 33, 36, 122, 125

delusions, 32, 33, 36, 85, 121, 123, 124, 125, 126, 127

denial, 19, 30, 117

depression, ix, x, 13, 19, 21, 28, 29, 35, 37

differentiation, 31, 35, 43, 59, 60, 67, 72, 73, 74, 86, 123, 124

discharge, 9, 19, 23, 24, 25, 52, 57, 60, 67, 68, 69, 70, 71, 91, 101

displacement, 19, 58, 59, 60, 62, 75, 113, 119

distortion, 58, 59, 60, 61, 62, 72, 75

dream, 6, 23, 43, 46, 47, 48, 50, 51, 52, 53, 54, 55, 56, 57, 58, 59, 60, 61, 62, 63, 64, 73, 75, 77, 97, 98, 99, 100, 101, 102, 103, 104, 105, 106, 108, 109, 113, 114, 120, 121, 123

ego strength, 19, 23, 24, 25, 30, 36, 37, 74, 78, 104, 105, 106, 118, 119, 120, 123

emotion, 4, 5, 8, 9, 10, 27, 43, 80, 81, 120